Essential Oils for Soothing Anxiety

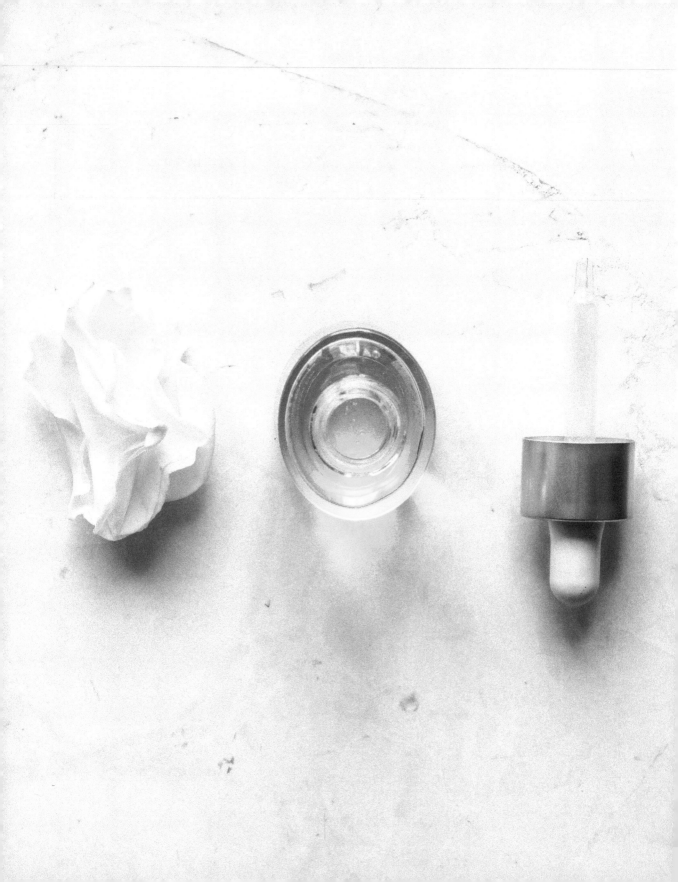

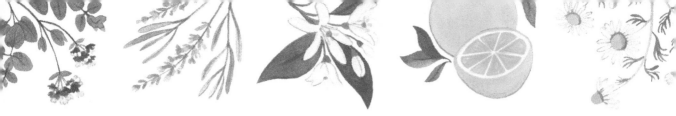

ESSENTIAL OILS
for Soothing Anxiety

Remedies and Rituals to Feel Calm and Refreshed

CHRISTINA ANTHIS

ROCKRIDGE
PRESS

Interior and Cover Designer: Stephanie Mautone
Art Producer: Sara Feinstein
Editor: Samantha Barbaro
Production Editor: Ruth Sakata Corley
Photography © 2019 Helene Dujardin, cover; Nadine Greeff/Stocksy, p. ii, v, 9, 132; Katarina Radovic/Stocksy, p. vi, 13; Ruth Black/Stocksy, p. viii, 23, 35, 59, 77, 97, 109, 131; Alicia Bock/Stocksy, p. x-1, 26-37.
Illustration © Kelsey Garrity-Riley, p. iii, 2, 6, 14, 20, 24-34, 38, 60, 78, 98, 110.
Author photo courtesy of © Brittany Carmichael.

ISBN: 978-1-64611-488-7 | eBook 978-1-64611-489-4
R0

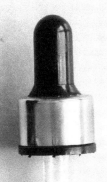

To my parents, who have always been my #1 fans, best friends, and biggest supporters throughout my life. I love you guys!

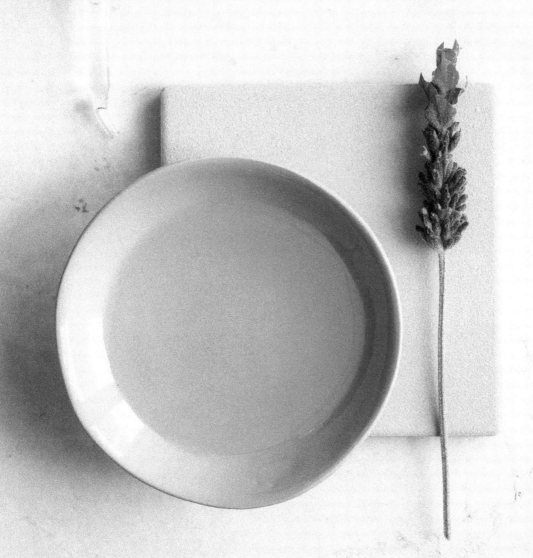

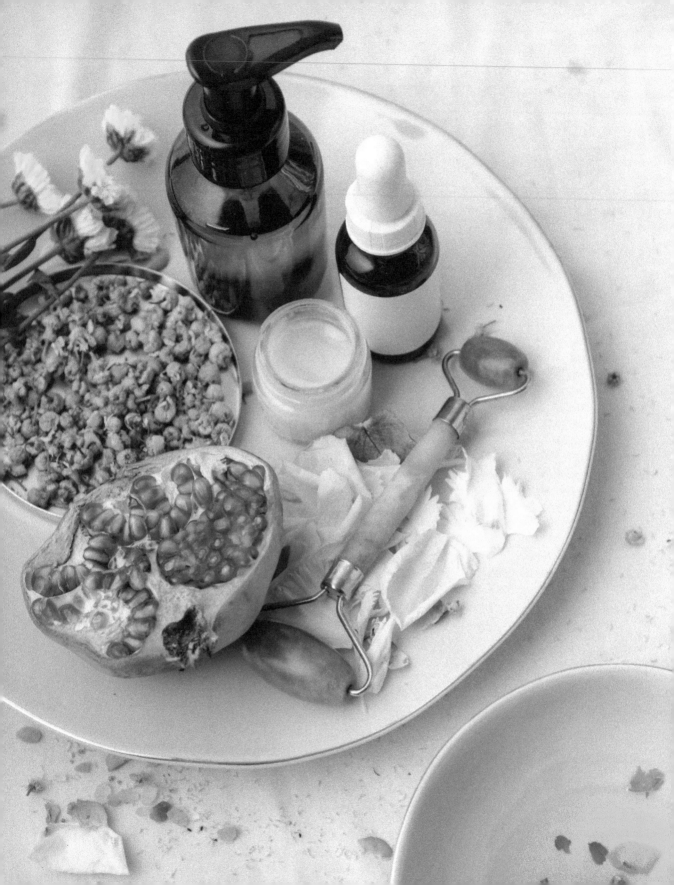

Contents

Introduction

I am often referred to as "smiley," "outgoing," and "happy," but these descriptions reflect masks I wear in public. What most people don't see are my moments of depression, anxiety, and even pain. We all carry these burdens. It's not how we carry them that matters, though; it's what we do to make them lighter that is most important.

A decade ago, just before I began my certification studies into aromatherapy and herbalism, I was feeling these burdens, but I didn't know how to fix them. It wasn't until after I started writing my blog, TheHippyHomemaker.com, that I really learned the importance of self-care.

As I started making and sharing aromatherapy recipes for relaxation, meditation, and natural health, I found myself taking time to use those recipes—and do you know what happened? I started to feel better. I was less anxious, my aches and pains were less frequent, and my immune system grew stronger. Once I made the connection between my emotional well-being and my physical health, I started making time to implement rituals and practices that helped me cope with all the emotions I was experiencing daily.

Essential oils have played a huge role in my journey to health, helping calm my mind when I couldn't sleep, relax my nerves from stage fright, and even soothe my emotions when frustration and sadness threatened to overwhelm me. Essential oils can help with a variety of issues, including stress, tension, insomnia, headaches, and much more.

My intentions with this book are to give you the tools and information you need to use essential oils for anxiety, stress, depression, and all the symptoms that can come with emotional distress. In part 1, I explain how you can benefit from using essential oils, how to use them safely, and the science behind their effectiveness. In addition, I will introduce you to self-care rituals and practices you can use alongside the recipes in this book. These practices include breathing techniques, meditations, and massage exercises. I will also delve deeper into my top 10 essential oils for calming and relaxation, their safety profiles, and many uses.

Part 2 comprises five chapters filled with aromatherapy recipes and corresponding rituals. You will find information on relaxation, breathing, meditation, restoring your sense of well-being, and remedies for everything from headaches to stomach upset. You will learn how to make soothing self-care products, how to increase your focus through breathing, how to relax your mind and body to release tension, how to use essential oils with reflexology and massage, and much more.

Whether you are looking for simple recipes to ease stress after a long day, or you want remedies that will help support you through the tougher times, I hope this book will become a valuable tool in your self-care library.

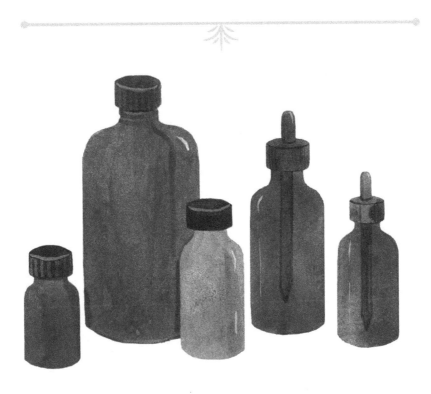

PART ONE

Essential Oils for Peace and Calm

For centuries essential oils have bridged the gap between ancient medicine and modern science, but it's only now, during the twenty-first century, that science has started uncovering what our ancestors already knew: Essential oils are more than just lovely fragrances.

In part 1, I offer an in-depth introduction to essential oils, starting with how they are extracted, the history and science behind them, and how to use them safely, whether through inhalation or topical applications. Then in part 2, I introduce you to the rituals and practices that appear throughout the book. When used in combination with the recipes, these healing rituals can help calm the nerves and soothe an uneasy mind. Finally, I provide 10 in-depth profiles of key essential oils for calming, relaxation, and more.

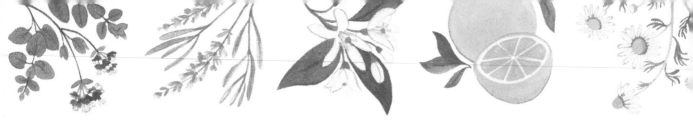

1

All About Essential Oils

Sometimes the demands of a fast-paced world can run a person ragged. In those times, especially, it is important to "stop and smell the roses." Literally. Although this expression implies slowing down and relaxing, the act of breathing in that subtle fragrance allows you to experience the calming benefits of the rose's essential oils.

Essential oils are volatile aromatic compounds produced by plants to protect themselves, give them their distinctive scents, and aid in pollination. When inhaled, aromatic compounds can play an important role in supporting a sense of calm, as well as overall health and well-being.

In this chapter, we'll review essential oil basics: their history, related research, how the oils are extracted, and how to use them safely.

History

Although essential oils may seem like the latest natural health fad, they have actually been in use for thousands of years. The earliest known recorded evidence dates back to around 2500 BCE in Egypt, where aromatic oils were used in spiritual practices, for embalming, and as health and beauty aids.

Around the same time, ancient Indian doctors and healers were also using aromatic oils in Ayurveda, a form of holistic medicine still practiced in India today. Many other ancient cultures and religions, including the Greeks, Romans, Chinese, Jews, and Christians, all have recorded evidence of their use of aromatic oils in medicine, beauty, and home care.

In Europe during the Middle Ages, the Catholic Church denounced the use of aromatic oils and herbs as "witchcraft" and imposed harsh consequences on those who used them. In an ironic twist, many historians credit monks of that time with secretly keeping the wisdom of herbal medicine alive. Despite the censorship that occurred in the Middle Ages, however, the use of essential oils and herbs did not die out.

Essential Oils Today

In the 1800s, some medical texts in Europe discussed essential oils alongside pharmaceuticals, but it wasn't until 1910 that modern science started to recognize the healing properties of essential oils. That year, a lab explosion left René-Maurice Gattefossé, a renowned French perfume chemist, with severe chemical burns on his hands, which developed into a serious infection of gas gangrene. Gattefossé knew the chemical properties of lavender essential oil and guessed it would help heal the infection. He applied the essential oil to his sores and found that just one application of lavender essential oil completely stopped the "gasification of the tissue." Gattefossé then continued to research essential oils and used his knowledge to help treat soldiers in World War I. The anecdotal evidence he collected during the war served as the basis of his 1937 book, *Aromatherapie*, which was the first time the word "aromatherapy" was seen in print.

Gattefossé's findings were reinforced during World War II when another Frenchman, physician, and army surgeon, Jean Valnet, used essential oils to treat his patients. He subsequently wrote numerous definitive works on aromatherapy, and Western physicians began to recognize the medical benefits of essential oils.

In 1977 the leading expert in the science and safety of essential oil use, Robert Tisserand, published *The Art of Aromatherapy*, bringing aromatherapy into the spotlight. His later book *Essential Oil Safety: A Guide for Health Care Professionals* (2nd edition) set industry standards for documenting the safe and practical use of essential oils and was the first published review of essential oil–drug interactions. His book continues to be an indispensable resource, with nearly 4,000 citations and essential oil constituent data not currently found anywhere else.

Extraction Methods

Essential oils are produced by extracting volatile essences from the roots, leaves, fruits, and flowers of grasses, plants, and trees. The amount of plant matter needed to produce the essential oil varies and can affect the price, which is the reason some essential oils cost more than others.

Depending on which part of the plant is being used, there are several methods to extract essential oils:

* **Steam distillation.** The most common method of extraction, steam distillation is a process by which plant matter and water are combined and brought to a boil in a sealed pot. The resultant steam, a combination of essential oil and hydrosol, rises up and flows through a tube into a condenser where it is cooled. As the steam settles back into liquid form, the essential oils float on top of the hydrosol and can then be easily skimmed off and bottled.

* **Cold pressed.** The cheapest and easiest method of extraction, cold pressing is only used on the peels of citrus fruits, which are chopped and soaked in water, then pressed, causing the oil and water to separate. The essential oils floating on top of the water are skimmed off. (Note: Due to their chemical makeup, many citrus essential oils that are cold pressed instead of steam distilled can cause a rash-like reaction—called sensitization—on the skin when exposed to sunlight after application.)

* **Absolutes and CO_2 extracts.** When plant matter is too fragile to withstand distillation, solvent extraction is used. Solvent extraction uses a smaller amount of plant matter and is often used to create more affordable essential oils from delicate flowers, such as jasmine and rose. If you can't afford to purchase the more expensive steam-distilled versions of these oils, the absolute oil works just as well and has many of the same healing properties.

Why Use Essential Oils?

If you are new to aromatherapy, it might be surprising to learn there are many ways beyond a diffuser that essential oils can be used. Every essential oil has its own set of properties, making it great for many different applications. Some of these beneficial properties include being antibacterial, antifungal, anti-inflammatory, analgesic, anti-depressant, and more.

Essential oils can be used for a variety of purposes:

* **Physical health.** When exhaustion and stress set in and illness threatens, essential oils are handy tools to have on your shelf. Highly antibacterial essential oils, such as cinnamon, lavender, oregano, and tea tree, can be used to support the immune system, whereas other essential oils, such as eucalyptus, fir needle, peppermint, and rosalina, can be used to help you breathe easier. One of my favorite and most versatile essential oils, sweet marjoram, can be used for immune support and easier breathing; plus it reduces pain and helps relax the body for sleep.

* **Natural beauty.** We're all looking to reduce fine worry lines, wrinkles, and acne, but the many beauty products that purport to transform our skin can be costly. What would you think if I said you can easily make your own natural beauty products at a fraction of the cost using essential oils? Many essential oils have skin-healing properties that make them perfect for soothing skin conditions, putting moisture back into dry skin, and even reducing wrinkles and fine lines. Some of my favorite skin-healing essential oils include chamomile, frankincense, lavender, and rose.

* **Mental health.** Stress is a common factor in all our lives. It can affect your mood, focus, immunity, and the ability to get quality sleep. When stress and anxiety are affecting your ability to cope, essential oils such as lavender, chamomile, clary sage, and grapefruit can ease tension and calm the nerves. In fact, lavender is such a powerhouse essential oil it can be used to calm a restless mind at bedtime and even improve focus and memory during the day.

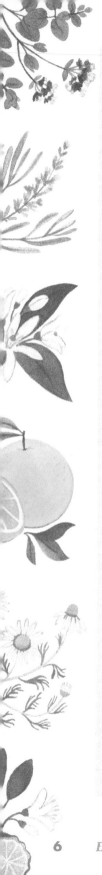

Your Essential Toolkit

If you are new to aromatherapy, there are a few ingredients and tools to keep on hand to make the remedies in this book.

Ingredients in This Book

Bath salts. Although there are many types of salt that can be used in the bath recipes in this book, Epsom salt is my favorite because it's rich in magnesium.

Beeswax. Beeswax is often used in cosmetic applications to harden or thicken a final product.

Healing clays. Especially beneficial in facial care, skincare, and hair care, healing clays are a natural beauty staple.

Shea butter. Shea butter is a key ingredient in many skincare applications, including body butter, skin-healing salves, soap, and moisturizing creams.

Witch hazel extract. This antiseptic extract is derived from the bark of the witch hazel tree. It is often used as a gentler alternative to alcohol and is my favorite choice in all skincare applications.

Tools to Get Started Using Essential Oils

Aromatherapy inhalers. Small in size and for personal use only, aromatherapy inhalers make on-the-go inhalation easy.

Assorted specialty bottles (⅓ ounce to 8 ounces). One-third-ounce roll-on bottles make topical application a breeze. Other bottles that are handy to have include spray or pump-top bottles, lotion pump bottles, and flip-top bottles.

Dark glass essential oil bottles. You need empty essential oil bottles when mixing undiluted essential oil blends, and dark glass helps protect the delicate oils from sunlight's potentially deteriorating effects.

Electric diffusers. A good diffuser is a must-have tool in your home. There are several types of aromatherapy diffusers on the market, but I prefer ultrasonic diffusers.

Jewelry diffusers. The new craze, jewelry diffusers are great for on-the-go diffusion and can complement your style, too!

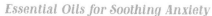

Essential Safety

One of the most important issues when working with essential oils is safety. Even though essential oils come from natural sources, that does not mean they are automatically without side effects, risks, or adverse reactions. When used incorrectly, essential oil injuries can and do occur. Some essential oil injuries that have been reported include rashes and burns on the skin, lesions in the mouth and throat, stomach ulcers, and even damage to the liver. These injuries can easily be avoided by adhering to the following basic essential oil safety guidelines.

Dilution

Dilution is the key to safety when using essential oils topically. Never apply essential oils directly on the skin (or "neat") without a carrier oil to dilute it. Some essential oils can cause irritation to the skin if they are not diluted sufficiently.

Oils that produce a warming or burning sensation when applied to the skin ("hot oils"), such as black pepper, cinnamon, clove, marjoram, nutmeg, and peppermint, should be highly diluted to prevent skin irritation. But even gentler oils, such as lavender and tea tree oils, should be diluted.

By using any essential oil neat on the skin, you risk developing a sensitization, or allergy, to that essential oil, which can be permanent. In her book, *Essential Oils and Aromatics*, Marge Clarke warns of this problem. "One of my mentors reminds me 'sensitization is forever.' . . . Years ago . . . I very unwisely used undiluted lavender on broken skin and, consequently, set up a sensitivity reaction. Today, almost two decades later, if I come in contact with lavender in any form, I will immediately start a new round of contact dermatitis that can take months to heal."

In his book, *Essential Oil Safety* (2nd edition), Robert Tisserand strongly recommends diluting essential oils "to avoid skin reactions," further adding that "skin reactions are totally dilution-dependent, and safety guidelines exist to minimize the risk."

The good news is dilution is as easy as combining essential oils with a carrier oil. The dilution percentage depends on the type of application, who the application is for, and the age of the person it will be applied to. I have provided a basic dilution chart that is taught in aromatherapy practice (see page 10). It is important to keep in mind that this is a general reference chart for blends, but some essential oils require more dilution than others. So, educating yourself on each oil you use can help prevent any unforeseen reactions.

Carrier Oils

Often referred to as base oils or fixed oils, carrier oils are not the same as essential oils. Although essential oils are volatile (they evaporate) and extremely concentrated, carrier oils are base vegetable oils (many of which you probably have in your pantry) that are cold pressed and used to dilute and "carry" essential oils. They are often used in cosmetics for their moisturizing and healing properties, and in massage oils for their natural glide. Any lotion, butter, or soap you own contains some form of carrier oil in its ingredients list. Although there are many types of carrier oils, the following list details my six favorites, which I keep on hand for all my aromatherapy needs:

1. **Avocado seed oil.** We know how healthy avocados are, but their awesome benefits don't stop with just eating them. Easy to find at the grocery store, refined avocado oil has little to no smell, a clear color, and it is deeply moisturizing to dry skin and hair. I love to use avocado oil in facial moisturizers, hair conditioners, and whipped body butters. Avocado oil is a heavier oil, meaning it sinks in slowly making it great for moisturizing applications.

2. **Coconut oil.** One of my favorite oils, I could write an entire book on coconut oil, and others already have. In its unrefined state, it hardens in temperatures colder than 76°F, making it a favorite of mine for simple salves. Naturally antibacterial, antifungal, antiseptic, and anti-inflammatory, coconut oil is healing and soothing to the skin and can even be applied to cuts and scrapes with lavender essential oil, as a simple "ouch" antibacterial cream.

3. **Fractionated coconut oil** does not harden like unrefined coconut oil and has no smell, making it a great carrier oil to use in essential oil roll-on applications. Coconut oil can be a tad on the dry side and is fairly comedogenic, meaning it can clog your pores. I suggest avoiding it in facial oils and moisturizers, but it's fantastic for all other applications.

4. **Grapeseed oil.** Grapeseed oil is rich in the same antioxidants found in wine. This natural anti-inflammatory oil has little to no scent and is one of the best oils to use in aromatics because it carries scents for long periods. It is great for perfume-type blends and aromatherapy roll-ons. I frequently use this oil in my facial oil, salves, and in a DIY scar cream. Grapeseed oil sinks into the skin quickly and is non-comedogenic.

5. **Hemp seed oil.** One of the best carrier oils to combat acne, hemp seed oil is rated the lowest on the comedogenic scale, meaning it's the oil least likely to clog your pores. This oil is one of my favorite oils to use in my facial oils and

moisturizers, body butter, and lotions because it sinks in quickly and leaves my skin feeling extremely soft. Hemp seed oil has a nutty scent that can overpower essential oils when not combined with other carrier oils.

6. **Olive oil.** As a Greek, I keep olive oil as a staple carrier oil in my home. Rich in antioxidants and healing and nourishing to the skin, olive oil is great for many applications. Growing up, we used olive oil to moisturize our faces, condition our hair, and even fix a squeaky door. Now I love to use this oil in all my healing salves. Naturally antibacterial, olive oil mixes well with coconut oil to make herbal-infused oils for skin-healing salves and lip balms. Extremely moisturizing but a bit greasy, this oil works well by itself but is even better mixed with another carrier oil. Olive oil has a nutty scent that can take over the scent of a blend, if not mixed with another carrier oil.

Note: If you have a nut allergy, avoid using nut oils and coconut oil to prevent an allergic reaction. All the other carrier oils suggested here are nut-allergy friendly, but you still may want to avoid the coconut oil.

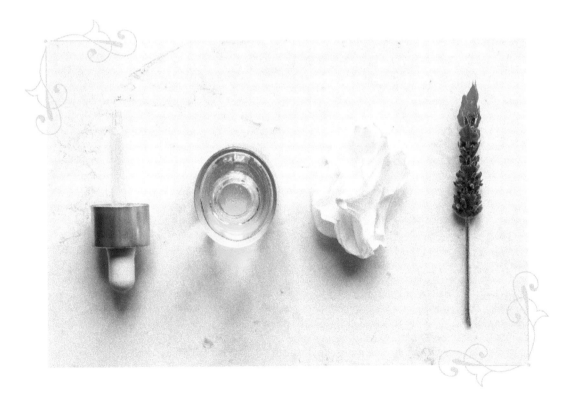

TRADITIONAL DILUTION CHART

CARRIER OIL	0.5%	1%	1.5%	2.5%	3%	5%	10%
½ ounce	1 or 2 drops	3 drops	5 drops	7 or 8 drops	9 drops	15 drops	30 drops
1 ounce	3 drops	6 drops	9 drops	15 drops	18 drops	30 drops	60 drops
2 ounces	6 drops	12 drops	18 drops	30 drops	36 drops	60 drops	120 drops

DILUTION	USES
0.5%	Babies, frail/elderly individuals
1%	Babies, children, pregnancy/nursing, frail/elderly individuals
1.5%	Subtle aromatherapy, emotional and energetic work, pregnancy/nursing, frail/elderly individuals, face creams, lotions, exfoliants
2.5% to 3%	Massage oils, general skincare, lotions, facial oils, body oils, body butter
5%	Treatment massages, acute treatment, wound healing, healing salves, body butter
10%	Muscular aches and pains, trauma injury, treatment massage, acute physical pain, salves and balms

Safe Dosage

To be on the safe side, essential oils should always be used as minimally as possible. I always start with the smallest dose and increase it based on the severity of the issue. Safe dosages are dependent on the type of application, who is using it, the user's age, and the reason for application.

There are many ways to apply essential oils, but the two safest modes are topical application and inhalation. Topical applications require dilution with a carrier oil to be deemed safe (see Traditional Dilution Chart, page 10).

Inhalation is the safest type of application when using essential oils. Simply follow the directions that come with your essential oil diffuser (use half the number of drops and half the diffusing time for pregnant women, babies, and children), and set your diffuser to 30 minutes on, 30 minutes off to prevent headaches or overexposure.

Topical Application

Topical application is a very common way to use essential oils, but requires dilution to be safe. This method of use can include both external skin and the linings of the mouth, nose, and ears. Topical application is commonly used to treat the skin itself, using salves and creams to heal acne, eczema, psoriasis, cuts, scrapes, and more. Topical application can also be used as in a chest rub to soothe a cough and ease congestion, in massage oil for muscle pains, and in a soothing salve to relieve menstrual cramps. Although topical application is great for skin conditions and other issues, it is the slowest and most diluted way to get essential oils into your bloodstream. The rate of absorption is dependent on the thickness of the skin the oil is applied to and dilution of the cream, salve, or oil mixture.

Phototoxicity

Some essential oils should not be used topically before going out into sunlight or sunbathing or tanning, as they can cause a phototoxic reaction to the skin, which means you may get a red rash around the area of application. The phototoxic reaction occurs if you use certain cold-pressed citrus essential oils on your skin, with the exception of products that wash off in the shower, such as body wash and shampoo, before exposing your skin to the sun's rays, or the UV lights used in tanning beds. You do not need very many drops of some of these essential oils to see this reaction occur, whereas others can safely be used in small-percentage dilutions without any issues.

CITRUS ESSENTIAL OILS KNOWN TO BE PHOTOTOXIC

* Bergamot essential oil

* Bitter orange essential oil (cold pressed)

* Clementine essential oil

* Grapefruit essential oil

* Lemon essential oil (cold pressed)

* Lime essential oil (cold pressed)

* Mandarin leaf oil

NON-PHOTOTOXIC CITRUS ESSENTIAL OILS

* Bergamot essential oil FCF (also known as bergaptene free)

* Lemon essential oil (steam distilled only)

* Lemon leaf oil

* Lime essential oil (steam distilled only)

* Mandarin essential oil

* Orange leaf oil

* Sweet orange essential oil

* Tangelo essential oil

Inhalation

Inhalation is one of the most effective and popular methods of using essential oils. Essential oils are made up of a combination of chemical constituents. When inhaled these constituents travel to your brain, your lungs, or both. Though it is one of the oldest methods of drug use, inhalation has only recently been rediscovered in the pharmaceutical industry. One of the latest drugs to be used via olfaction is insulin. Essential oils can be used through inhalation, in a variety of ways and for a variety of reasons. Inhalation is commonly used for respiratory tract infections, allergies, headaches, asthma, prevention of illness, anxiety, depression, fatigue, nausea, insomnia, nicotine withdrawal, ADHD, and even PTSD.

> *Note: Just like any powerful synthetic pharmaceuticals, essential oils should only be ingested under the guidance of a medical practitioner, certified in clinical aromatherapy. In* Essential Oil Safety (2nd edition) *Tisserand writes, "only practitioners who are qualified to diagnose, trained to weigh risks against benefits, and have knowledge of essential oil pharmacology should prescribe essential oils for oral administration."*

Now that you know the basics of essential oils, you can start using essential oils to create a peaceful and calming environment in your own home. In the next chapter, I'll show you how to combine essential oils with self-care practices and exercises that will help you de-stress, relax, and even boost your energy.

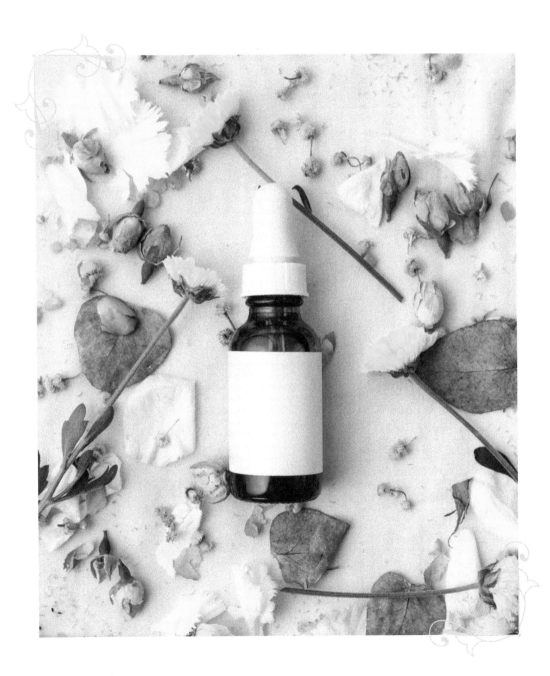

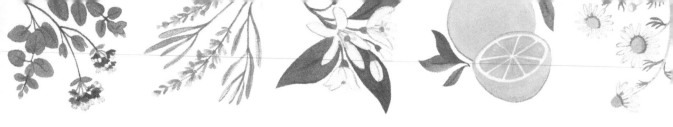

2

A Holistic Approach to Finding Peace and Calm

Lavender essential oil can bring peace and calm to any environment, but did you know the soothing scent of lavender combined with a basic breathing exercise can greatly reduce feelings of anxiousness, hyperventilation, and even panic? In this chapter, you will learn which essential oils have calming properties and how to combine them with self-care practices, breathing exercises, meditation, and massage to get the most effective results.

Holistic Healing

There is no one-size-fits-all cure for stress and anxiety. That's why it is important to focus on a holistic healing approach—looking at the body as a whole rather than focusing on isolated symptoms.

Stress can have diverse causes and equally diverse physical, mental, and emotional effects, but once you begin looking at your health from a big-picture perspective, you will start to see how physical and emotional well-being are connected. For this reason, this book emphasizes holistic self-care and combines calming essential oil remedies with meditation, focus on breath, and massage. Using these tools can help you find and maintain peace and calm in your day-to-day life.

The Research

Through anecdotal evidence, we've known for centuries that essential oils can help calm the mind and soothe the body, but it is only within the last 100 years that science has focused its magnifying glass upon essential oils and their many benefits.

In a 2015 study published in the *Journal of Caring Sciences*, researchers found that lavender essential oil is effective at significantly reducing stress, anxiety, and depression in pregnant patients, and a 2016 study in the *Journal of Clinical Anesthesia* showed that lavender oil had similar benefits in preoperative patients, and even ambulatory patients. A 2016 study in the journal *Phytotherapy Research* shows that certain citrus essential oils, including bergamot and sweet orange, can calm the nerves and soothe anxiety in cancer patients. Furthermore, a 2017 study in *MedSurg Nursing* even demonstrated the effectiveness of aromatherapy at reducing stress and anxiety in hospital nurses, whose job is known to entail high levels of stress.

Lavender, sweet orange, and laurel leaf essential oils have proved to alleviate symptoms of anxiety, stress, ADHD, PTSD, and even depression. As the science of aromatherapy keeps moving forward, modern medicine and essential oils will eventually become synonymous.

Soothing Essential Oils

There are a variety of essential oils with the ability to relax the body, alleviate stress, and even boost energy levels, but you don't need a vast collection of expensive oils to get results.

For this book, I have selected my "top 10" essential oils for finding peace and calm. These 10 essential oils will be used in many of the recipes and have a wide range of benefits aimed particularly at relieving anxiety, emotional distress, and related symptoms. I chose these oils, primarily, for their calming and soothing properties but also to provide the broadest benefits at a reasonable cost.

Here are my top 10 essential oils for helping you feel calm (you can find a more detailed profile of each oil in chapter 3):

1. **Bergamot.** This citrus-scented essential oil is well known for its ability to calm a restless mind at bedtime and soothe a nervous child. Like lavender essential oil, it has been studied extensively for its abilities to relieve stress, anxiety, and depression. Bergamot can aid digestion, stimulate the immune system, and even reduce headaches.

2. **Cedarwood.** Woody and grounding by nature, cedarwood essential oil has long been used by Native Americans to calm muscle spasms and aid the body in sleep. Cedarwood helps calm and focus the mind on the task at hand. It can also quiet an overactive mind at night. The woodsy scent of cedarwood is so calming that many find it works better for them than lavender. Together, they are unstoppable!

3. **Chamomile.** Everyone knows about the calming effects of chamomile herbal tea at bedtime, but the essential oil is even more powerful than the tea. Chamomile essential oil has the ability to help calm a child during a full-on tantrum, soothing their frazzled nerves and lulling them to sleep. Both blue chamomile and Roman chamomile essential oils are very gentle and soothing and are safe options for babies, children, and breastfeeding women.

4. **Coriander.** Rich in linalool, the same constituent found in lavender essential oil, coriander essential oil relaxes the mind and body. Recently studied in combination with lavender to help patients experiencing extreme anxiety, insomnia, and depression, coriander essential oil proved to be more effective at relieving symptoms than placebos and diazepam, an antianxiety drug. This citrus-scented essential oil has long been one of my personal favorite scents.

5. **Frankincense.** It's no wonder frankincense is mentioned in the bible as a gift: It's useful for so many things. Its earthy notes work well in any sleep blend, but it's also an immune support powerhouse, and can help soothe a headache. This grounding, earthy-scented resin has natural anti-inflammatory and antiseptic properties making it a go-to oil in skincare and wound healing, too. Like lavender, frankincense essential oil can pretty much do it all.

6. **Geranium.** Well known for its abilities to mitigate hormonal mood swings, geranium essential oil is an uplifting oil with a fragrant floral scent. This oil is often used to help balance hormones during menstruation and can help reduce cramps when applied to the abdomen in combination with a heating pad.

7. **Grapefruit.** This essential oil's uplifting citrus scent mixes well with all oils and is always a great top note to add a dash of happiness to an essential oil blend. Grapefruit essential oil has antidepressant, antibacterial, and digestive properties. In studies, grapefruit essential oil has been shown to reduce anxiety, quell a bad mood, and even alleviate premenstrual symptoms.

8. **Lavender.** The ultimate feel-good essential oil, everyone knows lavender is great at calming and soothing even the youngest of children. But, did you know it's a natural analgesic, meaning it can relieve pain? Lavender essential oil is probably one of the most heavily studied essential oils in the industry and it has proved its worth time and again. Naturally anti-inflammatory, lavender essential oil can soothe sore muscles and help relieve stress before bedtime.

9. **Neroli.** Although this essential oil is slightly pricier than the others, it is the perfect gentle oil to keep on hand when you need a break from the world. This delightfully sweet and floral oil is distilled from orange blossoms and is often used for dealing with grief, nervous tension, or exhaustion. It is kid safe and an excellent companion to chamomile essential oil in the kids' playroom.

10. **Sweet Marjoram.** Though this essential oil doesn't get as much credit as some others, marjoram essential oil is one of my personal favorites to keep on hand because it's so multi-faceted and always useful for bringing peace when I'm at my wit's end. Well known for its antispasmodic and anti-inflammatory properties, marjoram is often used for relieving muscle pain, tension, and even headaches, but it also has antianxiety benefits that make it a wonderful addition to any calming blend—I love it blended with lavender and coriander.

You Might Feel...

Stress and anxiety can cause a variety of physical and emotional symptoms, and they may not be the same for each individual. You may feel symptoms of fatigue, insomnia, high blood pressure, restlessness, difficulty concentrating, irritability, muscle tension, or a combination of these and other symptoms. With this in mind, I include remedies here for all the symptoms you might experience so you can focus on the specific issues affecting you.

A Complement to Conventional Medicine

As a lover of science, I want to note that the remedies in this book are not meant to substitute for the current medications you might be taking, or your doctor's advice. All the remedies in this book were created to complement conventional medicine, and I have taken the care to mention precautions or potential interactions with each essential oil used in these remedies.

Please consult your physician before making any changes to your medical routines and understand that although essential oils can be very effective at relieving stress and anxiety, they likely cannot do the job alone. If you are struggling with depression, anxiety, or PTSD, it is important that you visit a mental health professional for diagnosis and treatment. Essential oils can be used along with conventional medicine to alleviate symptoms and side effects you might be experiencing.

Although most essential oil creations will not have adverse reactions, some essential oils can conflict with certain medications. If you are currently taking medications of any sort, check with your doctor to be sure none of the oils you're using can interact negatively with your medicine. You can find more information on this topic in Tisserand's book, *Essential Oil Safety* (2nd edition), in which he lists essential oil–drug interactions for each individual essential oil that has been currently studied.

Rituals in This Book

This book is different from my other essential oil books because it pairs complementary rituals with essential oil recipes to help you build a stronger, more positive connection between your mind and body. These calming rituals include self-care practices, breathing exercises, meditation, and mantras as well as reflexology and massage. Although you can use any recipe in this book without the rituals and practices—and vice versa—using these tools together can help bring you a greater sense of well-being and inner peace.

Self-Care

It wasn't until my late 20s that I really began to appreciate the benefits of self-care. Before that, I was running myself into the ground at full speed. I used to look at self-care as a luxury and not something everyone needs to maintain a healthy equilibrium. I didn't realize my batteries were being depleted and I wasn't taking time to recharge them. Now I know: Self-care is important. When you begin practicing self-care, you will see a significant difference in how you feel mentally, physically, and emotionally.

Self-care can look different for different people because each individual has different mental, emotional, and physical needs. For some, self-care may be getting a full eight hours of sleep at night, whereas for others it might be taking time to acknowledge and process the feelings felt throughout the day. One day you may need a muscle-soothing bubble bath with a side of music, whereas another day you might require complete silence and a moment to breathe. This book focuses on self-care in many different forms to help you get beyond just coping and into the practice of giving yourself what you need to live peacefully on a day-to-day basis.

If you are new to self-care and want to start with the basics, chapter 4 is a great place to begin. There you will find a variety of natural beauty and self-care remedies that will help you create the feel of a relaxing spa environment in your own home.

A Soothing Space

One important component of finding peace and calm in your daily life is to create a soothing space for relaxation, meditation, and calming rituals. This can look different for each individual and you can easily work with what you have available. A soothing space can help your brain focus faster, ease tension, and signal your body that it's time to let go and relax. Some things to think about when creating your soothing space include:

Lighting. Too much light streaming in can hinder your ability to focus during deep meditation. If you aren't able to shut curtains or dim the lights, a salt lamp might be a good option to light your soothing space gently. When I need darkness on the go, I pull out a sleep mask to cover my eyes and help me focus.

Pillows. In my opinion, no soothing space should be without pillows. You can use them to prop up your head when lying down or to support you while sitting upright.

Diffuser. What soothing aromatherapeutic space would be complete without a diffuser? It's the cheapest and easiest method of using essential oils in your soothing space.

Temperature. Temperature can affect your ability to focus. I like to keep my home cool, but I always keep a blanket on hand in the event I get too cold while meditating.

Music. Music doesn't have to be in your soothing space, but it's always included in mine. No matter your tastes in music, it has a proven ability to affect your mood and has been clinically proven to increase focus and stimulate meditative states in the brain, making it easier for you to slip into a relaxed and happy place.

Listen to Your Breath

The practice of mindful breathing is shared by many cultures and groups around the world and across time, including in ancient warrior traditions and with Buddhists, as well as among yoga and qigong practitioners. The Navy SEALs teach their soldiers breathing techniques to use in situations where panic might get in the way of action. Breathing exercises can improve health, focus the mind, help control physical responses, and improve performance under pressure. Any breathing exercise in this book can be used to help you calm your emotions, stop a panic attack, and even help your brain function better when working in tense situations.

Be with Your Thoughts

Meditation can reduce stress levels, reduce pain, increase cognitive function, improve moods, and combat depression. During meditation, your brain achieves deeper states of relaxation than it does during sleep. Just 5 to 10 minutes of meditation a day can positively affect your well-being. That means that even if you "don't have time," you still have time.

Over the last 60 years, tons of studies have confirmed the numerous benefits of meditation. Meditation has been shown to:

* Boost productivity

* Help overcome addiction

* Increase brain capacity, power, and function

* Increase compassion and love

* Increase memory and learning ability

* Increase self-esteem and self-awareness

* Lower blood pressure and cholesterol

* Make you happier

* Reduce anger and emotional instability

* Reduce inflammation and pain

* Relieve stress and calm anxiety

* Treat migraines and headaches

In chapter 6, I provide an assortment of meditations paired with aromatherapy remedies to help you learn how to find your Zen. With these easy-to-learn meditations, you can meditate no matter how busy life is. In combination with essential oils, meditation has the potential to improve your health and increase happiness.

Massage and Reflexology

Evolved from an ancient Chinese therapy, reflexology is, essentially, a system involving massage or a degree of pressure placed on certain areas of the body that is used to relieve tension, stress, anxiety, headaches, and even digestive upset. The practice is based on the theory that there are specific places called "reflex points" on the feet, hands, and other body areas linked to helping restore proper functioning of the body, increasing blood flow to the extremities, slowing heart rate, and decreasing blood pressure. This gentle therapy feels soothing to the nerves and has shown promising results in studies at helping patients relax and feel a sense of calm.

Although reflexology can help with many different conditions, it is especially effective for anxiety and its many different symptoms.

Combining calming rituals and essential oils is an effective form of holistic self-care that will help you achieve overall well-being. In the next chapter, I provide in-depth profiles of my top 10 essential oils for peace and calm. In each profile, you will find information on each essential oil, including safety recommendations, uses, applications, and more.

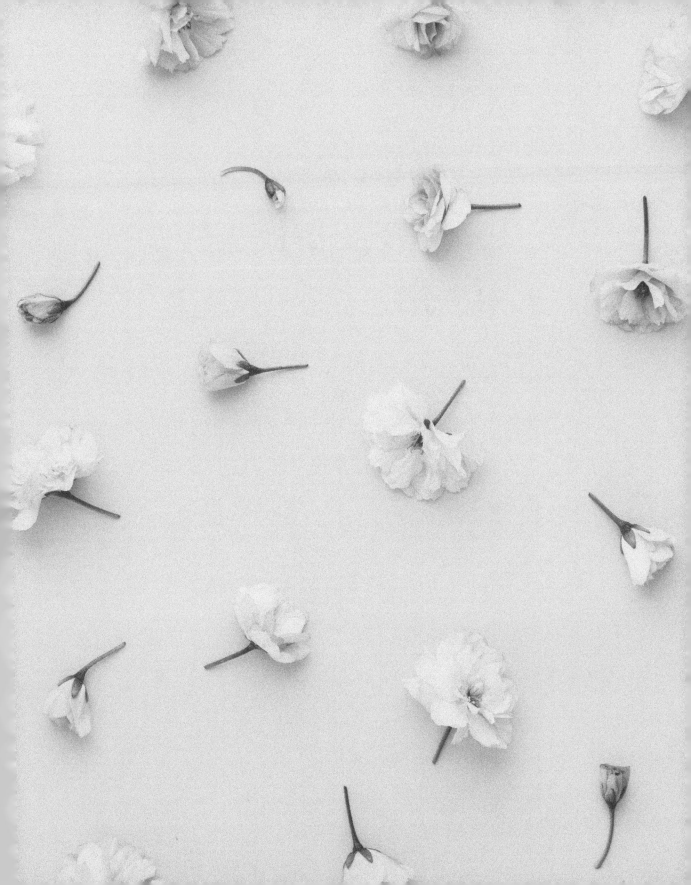

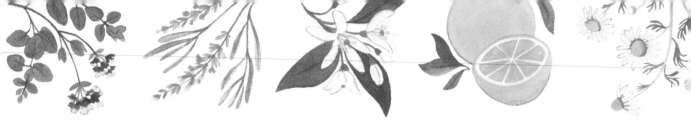

3

Key Essential Oils for Calming, Relaxation, and More

Bergamot, *Citrus bergamia*

Bergamot essential oil is a bright, citrusy-scented oil with a hint of floral spice that brings thoughts of happiness and peace during tough times. This unique and vibrant essential oil is well known for its ability to brighten your mood and ease your worries. Bergamot essential oil is often used to treat insomnia, depression, and anger.

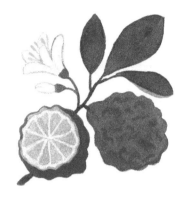

Precautions: For topical applications, look for bergaptene-free (FCF) bergamot essential oil to avoid phototoxicity from exposure to sunlight.

Benefits: Alleviates anxiety and depression symptoms; alleviates eczema and psoriasis symptoms; promotes hair growth, reduces indigestion and gas, relieves headaches and insomnia; relieves itching; soothes muscle aches and pains; treats acne

Best for: Anxiety, depression, digestive issues

Applications: Bergamot essential oil can be added to salves and massage oils to help relieve aching muscles, headaches, and indigestion. When added to skincare products, including salves, facial cleansers, toners, and moisturizers, bergamot can help cleanse and heal eczema and improve stress- and hormone-related skin conditions, like teenage acne. Bergamot is often used in diffuser blends, aromatherapy roll-ons, and shower steamers.

✳ Dilute 9 drops of bergamot essential oil in 1 ounce hemp seed oil to make an effective moisturizer for acne or oily skin. After cleansing your face, massage 1 or 2 drops in a circular motion over your entire face, or use as a spot treatment. Avoid getting the oil into your eyes or mouth.

✳ Add 5 to 10 drops of bergamot essential oil to your diffuser and diffuse throughout your home to boost the mood and freshen the air.

✳ Are you in need of a relaxing getaway from a bad mood? Try Mood Maestro Shower Steamers (page 41) and let yourself be transported to a happier place.

Cedarwood, *Atlas, Cedrus atlantica*

This smoky, balsamic-scented essential oil is distilled from the wood and sawdust of the Atlas cedar. It is slightly orange-yellow in color and has deep woody undertones, like a fresh forest after the rain. Cedarwood essential oil is said to be grounding and calming; it can relax tense muscles and soothe frazzled nerves.

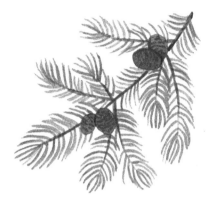

Precautions: None

Benefits: Aids meditation; calms hyperventilation and social anxiety; improves mental focus; relieves insomnia and nervous tension; soothes muscle aches and pains; soothes skin rashes, treats acne

Best for: ADHD/ADD, focus issues, insomnia

Applications: Cedarwood essential oil is often used in combination with lavender in the diffuser and aromatherapy roll-ons to help promote a sense of calm and focus or to relax the mind for sleep. When diffused in the office or classroom, cedarwood essential oil can increase mental focus, attentiveness, and improve test scores.

* Add 6 drops of Atlas cedarwood essential oil to a ⅓-ounce roll-on bottle and fill with fractionated coconut oil. Use to help with focus and meditation. Apply the roll-on behind the ears, on the back of the neck, and to the wrists before studying, practicing yoga, or meditating.

* Add 5 to 10 drops of cedarwood essential oil to your diffuser and diffuse throughout your home to ground and center your mind when you're having trouble focusing.

* Is panic making it hard for you to breathe? Try Panic Stopper Aromatherapy Inhaler (page 70) to help calm a panic attack.

Chamomile, *Roman, Anthemis nobilis or Chamaemelum nobile*

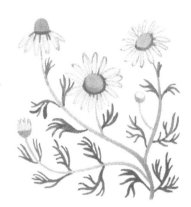

This sweet and charming floral essential oil has a calming, apple-like scent with soft herbaceous undertones. The essential oil is distilled from the daisy-like flowering tops of the plant and is pale yellow in color. Chamomile essential oil is well known for its gentle ability to calm fears in young children and help induce sleep.

Precautions: People with ragweed allergies should not use this essential oil.

Benefits: Alleviates anxiety and depression symptoms; alleviates menstrual cramps; calms anxious children; mitigates hormonal mood swings; reduces indigestion; relieves headaches, insomnia, and nervous tension; soothes muscle aches and pains; treats acne

Best for: Anxiety, digestive issues, insomnia, nervous tension

Applications: Roman chamomile essential oil is very gentle and can be used in a variety of topical applications, including healing salves, skincare, night creams, massage, and bedtime baths. Chamomile is also very therapeutic through inhalation when used in a diffuser, shower steamers, aromatherapy roll-ons, and personal inhalers.

❋ Are monsters in the closet keeping the kiddos up at night? Combine 20 drops lavender essential oil and 20 drops Roman chamomile essential oil in a 4-ounce spray bottle, then fill it with water. Cover and shake well before use. Spray the offending areas to calm your little one's fears so they can get a good night's rest!

❋ Add 10 drops chamomile essential oil to 1 ounce unscented bubble bath and pour under running bath water for a relaxing bedtime bath that's sure to soothe your mind and body for sleep.

❋ Trying to get to sleep but counting sheep isn't helping? Try Sleep Deep Massage Oil (page 100) to help calm your mind and body for a better night's rest.

Coriander, *Coriandrum sativum*

This bright, fruity essential oil is reminiscent of sweet citrus fruits with herbaceous undertones. Steam distilled from crushed coriander seeds, coriander essential oil is clear to pale yellow in color.

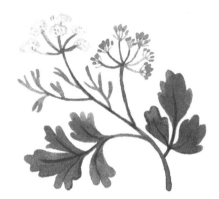

Precautions: None

Benefits: Alleviates anxiety and depression symptoms; alleviates eczema symptoms; alleviates menstrual cramps; calms; eases mental fatigue; induces relaxation; mitigates hormonal mood swings; provides immune support; reduces indigestion, inflammation, and stress; relieves insomnia, headaches, migraines, and nausea; soothes muscle aches and pains; stimulates appetite; treats acne

Best for: Depression, digestive issues, mental fatigue

Applications: Coriander essential oil is wonderful for a variety of applications. Coriander can be diluted in massage oil and massaged onto the abdomen to aid digestion. When coriander essential oil is added to diffuser blends, aromatherapy roll-ons, and shower steamers, it helps freshen the space and brighten the mood. If acne is a problem, coriander essential oil can help cleanse the skin and soothe inflammation.

* Dilute 15 drops of coriander essential oil in 1 ounce fractionated coconut oil for an after-dinner digestive tummy massage. Gently massage the oil onto your abdomen in a circular motion to relieve gas and indigestion.

* Add 5 to 10 drops of coriander essential oil to your diffuser and diffuse throughout your home to brighten the mood and help clear mental fog.

* Want to bring a little extra magic into your life? Try Rainbows and Unicorns Perfume Oil (page 63) to lighten the mood and bring a smile to your face.

Frankincense, *Boswellia carterii*

Used for thousands of years in incense and perfumery, frankincense essential oil works well during times of deep grief and sorrow. Steam distilled from African tree gum resin, this ancient essential oil works overtime to support the immune system, calm overactive nerves, and ground you during times of emotional upheaval.

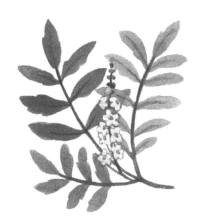

Precautions: None

Benefits: Aids meditation; alleviates anxiety symptoms; alleviates menstrual cramps; assuages grief and sadness; improves breath awareness and mental focus; mitigates hormonal mood swings; provides immune support; soothes muscle aches and pains; reduces indigestion and stress; relieves insomnia, nausea, nervous tension, and pain; treats acne

Best for: Anxiety, focus issues

Applications: Frankincense essential oil is a very useful essential oil that can be used in a variety of applications, including as salves for muscle pain, immune support, or hormonal fluctuations. When added to a diffuser, shower steam, or a personal inhaler, frankincense can help increase focus, improve cognitive function, calm the nervous system, and help you get to sleep.

✳ Add 6 drops of frankincense essential oil to a ⅓-ounce roll-on bottle and fill with fractionated coconut oil for help with focus and meditation. Apply the roll-on behind the ears, on the back of the neck, and to the wrists before studying, practicing breathing exercises, or meditating.

✳ Is your busy schedule getting in the way of your meditation practice? Try Instant Gratification Aromatherapy Inhaler (page 87) along with my 5-Minute On-the-Go Mantra Meditation (page 88). Even 5 minutes of meditation a day has been shown to improve cognitive function, reduce depression, and help support the body during stressful times.

Geranium, *Pelargonium x asperum, Pelargonium graveolens*

This essential oil is well known for its ability to help with women's menstrual pains and hormone-related mood swings; geranium is the oil you want on hand when Aunt Flo comes to town. Steam distilled from the leaves and flowers, this extremely floral-scented oil has sweet lemon and herbaceous undertones.

Precautions: None

Benefits: Alleviates anxiety and depression symptoms; alleviates eczema and psoriasis symptoms; alleviates menstrual cramps; eases mental fatigue; increases energy; mitigates hormonal mood swings; quells emotional outbursts; reduces anger and stress; relieves headaches, insomnia, and nervous tension; treats acne

Best for: Depression, hormonal fluctuations

Applications: Geranium essential oil is a wonderfully gentle essential oil that can be used in many different applications, including skincare, soothing lotions, aromatherapy roll-ons, and more! When added to your diffuser, geranium will help ease tension and stress in the home.

* Dilute 15 drops of geranium essential oil in 1 ounce fractionated coconut oil for a cramp-relieving massage. Gently massage the oil onto your abdomen in a circular motion to relieve menstrual cramps, calm frazzled nerves, and reduce bloating.

* Add 5 drops of geranium essential oil to your diffuser and diffuse throughout your home to soothe emotional upset and dispel negative feelings.

* Are feelings of anger and negativity keeping you down? Try using Open Your Heart Aromatherapy Roll-On (page 93) with the complementary Loving Kindness Meditation (page 94) to reduce anger and open yourself to joy.

Grapefruit, *Citrus paradisi*

Fruity and sweet, this fresh-smelling citrus essential oil is one of my favorites. Cold pressed from the peel of the grapefruit, grapefruit essential oil's joyful scent helps brighten the mood in any room by calming nervous tension and dispelling anger.

Precautions: Skin sensitization can occur if the oil is oxidized when used topically. Grapefruit essential oil is phototoxic if used at more than a 4 percent dilution, or 36 drops of essential oil per ounce of carrier oil. It is recommended to stay out of the sun for 12 hours after application if more than the maximum recommended dilution is used.

Benefits: Aids detoxification; alleviates anxiety and depression symptoms, assuages grief and sadness, elevates mood; increases energy; mitigates hormonal mood swings; promotes hair growth; provides immune support; reduces anger, stress, and indigestion; relieves headaches; suppresses appetite; treats acne

Best for: Acne, depression

Applications: When used in baths, creams, and salves, the scent of grapefruit essential oil can help assuage sadness. When added to a diffuser, grapefruit essential oil cleans and freshens the air with its sweet uplifting scent. It can also be used in face washes and toners to help clear breakouts on the skin.

* Add 10 drops grapefruit essential oil to 1 ounce unscented bubble bath and pour under running bath water for an energizing and uplifting start to your day.

* Add 10 drops of grapefruit essential oil to your diffuser and diffuse throughout your home for an energizing boost during the afternoon slump.

* Is your skin looking a bit dry in the middle of winter? Use Grapefruit Lavender Body Butter Bars (page 52) to moisturize your skin deeply during harsh winter months.

Lavender, *Lavandula angustifolia/officinalis*

One of the most popular essential oils, lavender can do almost any job. Although it is well known for its ability to calm a restless mind, lavender essential oil is most often used as a sleep aid and for pain relief. It can also help soothe your nerves when you are overstimulated. This sweet, floral-scented essential oil is steam distilled from the flowering tops of the plants.

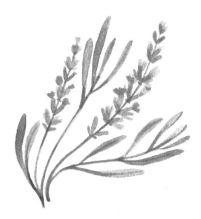

Precautions: None

Benefits: Alleviates anxiety symptoms; alleviates eczema symptoms; calms; improves attention and mental focus; reduces inflammation and stress; relieves headaches, insomnia, migraines, nausea, nervous tension, and pain; soothes muscle aches and pains; treats acne

Best for: Anxiety, insomnia, nervous tension, pain

Applications: Lavender essential oil can be used topically or through inhalation. There are a variety of ways to use lavender, including in salves, sprays, lotions or creams, baths, personal inhalers, and diffusers. Add lavender essential oil to a diffuser to help relieve stress, anxiety, and insomnia.

* Add 10 drops lavender essential oil to 1 ounce unscented bubble bath and pour under running bath water for a relaxing bedtime bath that also helps relieve achy, tense muscles.

* Diffuse 10 drops lavender essential oil in your bedroom at bedtime to calm a restless mind and help ease the body to sleep.

* Have the day's pressures given you a headache? Try using Headache Helper Roll-On (page 106) to soothe stress and tension headaches.

Marjoram, *Sweet, Majorana hortensis, Origanum majorana*

A well-known herb in the culinary world, this calming essential oil soothes achy muscles, digestive issues, and even headaches. When combined with lavender essential oil in a carrier, they relieve pains and spasms and soothe little ones to sleep. Steam distilled from the dried leaves and flowering tops of the plant, this woody herbaceous essential oil has warm, spicy, and camphorous aromas.

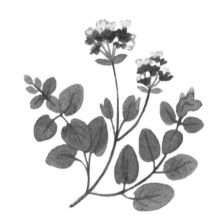

Precautions: Not to be confused with Spanish marjoram (*Thymus mastichina*), which has been shown to be toxic when taken orally and should not be used around children, the elderly, or pregnant or nursing women

Benefits: Alleviates anxiety symptoms and menstrual cramps; assuages grief and sadness; calms obsessive thinking; provides immune support; quells muscle spasms; reduces constipation, indigestion, and stress; relieves headaches, insomnia, nervous tension, pain, and restless leg syndrome; soothes muscle aches and pains

Best for: Digestive issues, insomnia, pain

Applications: Marjoram essential oil can be used in topical applications through massage, baths, salves, and skincare to help relieve pain, soothe frazzled nerves, and relax the body for sleep. Diffuse marjoram essential oil while meditating or before bed to calm the mind and help facilitate better breathing.

* Add 9 drops sweet marjoram essential oil to a ⅓-ounce roll-on bottle, then fill it with fractionated coconut oil for use as a soothing massage oil. Apply the roll-on to your legs and feet and massage it in to soothe restless legs.

* Add 5 to 10 drops sweet marjoram essential oil to your diffuser to support the immune system during times of high stress and tension.

* Try using Muscle Mender Bath Salts (page 39) to soothe muscle tension.

Neroli, *Citrus aurantium*

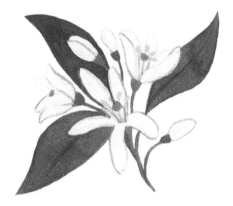

One of three essential oils deriving from the orange tree, neroli essential oil is made from orange blossoms. This sweet, delicate, floral essential oil naturally brightens the mood of any room, making it great for people dealing with grief, depression, or nervous tension. Neroli oil is also used in many skincare products for its ability to promote a healthy complexion.

Precautions: None known

Benefits: Alleviates anxiety and depression symptoms; assuages grief and sadness; improves mental focus; increases energy; mitigates hormonal mood swings; reduces anger and stress; relieves insomnia and nervous tension; treats acne

Best for: Depression, grief, nervous tension

Applications: Neroli essential oil can be used for topical applications through massage, baths, salves, and skincare. It is especially useful in facial creams and oils to help reduce scarring, wrinkles, and fine worry lines. This delightful essential oil can also be used in a diffuser or steam inhalation to cheer up and brighten the entire room.

* Combine 5 drops neroli essential oil and 4 drops coriander essential oil in a ⅓-ounce roll-on bottle, then fill with fractionated coconut oil to create a happy-scented perfume oil.

* Combine 3 drops neroli essential oil with 6 drops grapefruit in your diffuser to spread bright, uplifting cheer throughout your home.

* Try using Party Herbal Bath Tea (page 42) to relax and unwind from an especially stressful week.

PART TWO

Remedies and Rituals with Essential Oils

Essential oils can be used in a variety of ways to help treat the many symptoms that anxiety can produce. In this part, you will find essential oil blends, recipes, rituals, and techniques to help you relax, feel calm, and create a peaceful space.

This part begins with recipes for relaxing baths, shower steamers, body butter, and face masks to get you started on your self-care journey. In chapter 5, you will find remedies combined with easy breathing exercises to help calm the nerves and boost confidence. In chapter 6, you will learn just how easy it is to incorporate a meditative practice into your life—no matter how busy your schedule. Chapter 7 includes recipes for massage oils with instructions for short massages that will ease tension and release sore muscles. Finally, in chapter 8, I have included 20 on-the-spot treatments to address a wide range of anxiety-related symptoms, including headaches, nausea, and body aches.

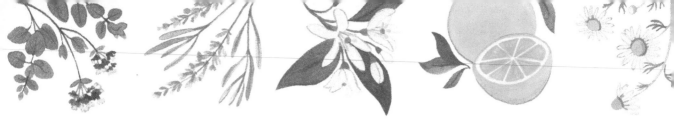

4

Relax

Muscle Mender Bath Salts

HEADACHES, MUSCLE ACHES, STRESS, TENSION • AROMATIC, TOPICAL • **MAKES 1 TREATMENT**

Safe for ages 2+ (use half the amount of essential oils for children 2 to 4 years of age)

This soothing muscle treatment is perfect after a long day of work, especially if your muscles are taxed or tense. Rich in magnesium, Epsom salt baths have been used alongside scented oils for centuries to supplement much-needed minerals in the body, soothe sore muscles, and promote healthier sleep. Rosalina essential oil, similar to lavender essential oil, helps relieve muscle tension and pain while washing away negative thoughts. Lavender essential oil helps calm frazzled nerves and soothes a harried mind, and marjoram essential oil relieves muscle pain and helps you let go of any worries from the day.

1. In a medium glass bowl, stir together the olive oil and rosalina, sweet marjoram, and lavender oils.

2. Using a spoon, stir the Epsom salt into the oil mixture.

3. Pour the mixture under running water as you fill the bathtub.

4. Soak in the tub for at least 20 minutes to feel the full benefits of this tension-relieving bath soak.

Helpful hint: *Don't want to deal with a slippery tub after the bath? Substitute your favorite unscented shampoo or bubble bath for the carrier oil in this recipe.*

2 tablespoons extra-virgin olive oil, or another liquid carrier oil

3 drops rosalina essential oil

3 drops sweet marjoram essential oil

3 drops lavender essential oil

1 cup Epsom salt

Spa Day Bubble Bath

ANXIETY, DEPRESSION, RELAXATION, STRESS • AROMATIC, TOPICAL • **MAKES 1 TREATMENT**

Safe for ages 2+ (use half the amount of essential oils for children 2 to 4 years of age); pregnant and nursing women should omit lemongrass essential oil

This relaxing bubble bath is designed to whisk you away from the cares and worries of the day and transform your bath into a calming spa retreat. The uplifting scents of citrus bliss will melt away your stress. For the ultimate spa experience, pair this bath with Bohemi Babe Herbal Mud Masks (page 44) and don't forget the final touch—organic cucumber slices for soothing your eyes.

1. In a medium glass bowl, stir together the bubble bath and coriander, bergamot, and lemongrass essential oils.

2. Using a spoon, stir the Dead Sea salt into the oil mixture.

3. Pour the mixture under running water as you fill the bathtub.

4. Soak in the tub for at least 20 minutes to feel the calming benefits of this spa-day bath.

2 tablespoons unscented bubble bath, or shampoo

4 drops coriander essential oil

3 drops bergamot essential oil

1 drop lemongrass essential oil

1 cup Dead Sea salt

Awesome addition: *Herbs such as lavender, chamomile, and mint make great additions to this bath. In a large cloth tea bag or an old sock, combine ¼ cup of each herb, dried, and tie the bag closed before tossing it into the bathtub. Note: If using fresh herbs, double the amounts.*

Mood Maestro Shower Steamers

DEPRESSION, EMOTIONAL UPHEAVAL, MENTAL FATIGUE, MOODINESS •
AROMATIC • **MAKES 6 TO 8 SHOWER STEAMERS**

Safe for ages 2+ (use half the amount of essential oils for children 2 to 4 years of age)

A centering aromatherapeutic shower steam is the perfect way to temper mood swings. These mood-elevating shower steamers will help soothe sadness and clear the mental fog on days when you feel like you're riding an emotional roller coaster. Pair your shower steam with music that makes you feel strong and grounded.

1. Wearing gloves and using your hands, in a medium glass bowl, combine the baking soda, citric acid, and cornstarch until there are no clumps remaining.

2. Add the bergamot, Atlas cedarwood, and grapefruit essential oils and, using your gloved hands, thoroughly mix them into the powders, breaking up small clumps.

3. Spray the mixture 2 or 3 times with witch hazel and continue to mix using your gloved hands until you can pack the mixture like a snowball without it crumbling. Repeat spraying the mixture if it is still too dry to hold together.

4. Pack the mixture into a ¼-cup measuring cup or silicone molds, pressing it in firmly. If using a measuring cup, gently turn the steamer out onto parchment paper or wax paper and let dry overnight. Repeat with the remaining mixture. If using silicone molds, let the steamers dry in the molds overnight before popping them out.

5. Keep the shower steamers in a sealed Mason jar, label and date your creation, and store in a cool, dark location.

6. To use, place one shower steamer at the end of the bathtub or shower, avoiding direct contact with the water. Let it slowly dissolve while you shower and breathe in the aromas.

1 cup baking soda

½ cup citric acid

1 tablespoon cornstarch, or arrowroot powder or any type of healing clay

½ teaspoon bergamot essential oil

25 drops Atlas cedarwood essential oil

25 drops grapefruit essential oil

Witch hazel, in a small spray bottle

Helpful hint: *If you get to the end of the batch of shower steamers and the scent has evaporated, add 5 drops of the essential oil blend used in the recipe to the tops of the shower steamers to refresh the scent before use.*

Party Herbal Bath Tea

ANXIETY, HEADACHES, INSOMNIA, STRESS • AROMATIC, TOPICAL • **MAKES 1 TREATMENT**

Safe for ages 2+ (use half the amount of essential oils for children 2 to 4 years of age)

What's more relaxing than a tea party in your bathtub? This tranquilizing herbal bath tea is designed to calm frazzled nerves, relieve tension, and help relax the body for bedtime. The soothing herbs and essential oils in this recipe are specifically chosen to help you let go after a hectic or stressful day. Sip a cup of lemon chamomile tea while you soak to complete the relaxing tea party in your tub!

1. In a medium glass bowl, stir together the carrier oil and chamomile, lavender, and sweet orange essential oils.

2. Using a spoon, stir the Epsom salt into the oil mixture.

3. Stir in the lavender buds, chamomile flowers, and lemon balm, stirring until combined.

4. Transfer the mixture to a cloth tea bag or an old sock and tie the bag closed before tossing it into a filled bathtub.

5. Soak in the tub for at least 20 minutes to feel the full effects of this soothing bath tea.

Did you know? *Herbal bath teas have been used for thousands of years for medicinal purposes. The ancient Greek physician Hippocrates developed hydropathy, a form of medical treatment using water. This treatment was passed along to Roman physicians and became in common use in the bathhouses of ancient Rome.*

2 tablespoons extra-virgin olive oil, or another liquid carrier oil

3 drops Roman chamomile essential oil

3 drops lavender essential oil

3 drops sweet orange essential oil

1 cup Epsom salt

¼ cup dried lavender buds

¼ cup dried chamomile flowers

¼ cup lemon balm

Island Getaway Hydrating Bath Bombs

DRY SKIN, NERVOUS TENSION, OVERSTIMULATION, STRESS •
AROMATIC, TOPICAL • **MAKES 8 TO 10 BATH BOMBS**

Safe for ages 2+ (use half the amount of essential oils for children 2 to 4 years of age)

When feeling overwhelmed and in need of escape, reach for these hydrating bath bombs to take you on a relaxing staycation. The tropical blend of essential oils will comfort an overstimulated body and help ease nervous tension, all while deeply moisturizing your skin. Enhance this bath with the soothing sounds of the ocean for a truly tropical experience.

1. Wearing gloves and using your hands, in a medium glass bowl, combine the baking soda, citric acid, coconut milk powder, and arrowroot powder until there are no clumps remaining.

2. In a small glass bowl, stir together the melted coconut oil and coriander, lime peel, ylang-ylang, and neroli essential oils until blended.

3. Pour the oil mixture into the powder mixture and mix well.

4. Spray the mixture 2 or 3 times with witch hazel and continue to mix, using your gloved hands, until you can pack the mixture into a snowball without it crumbling. Repeat spraying the mixture if it is still too dry to hold together.

5. Pack the mixture into a ¼-cup measuring cup or silicone molds, pressing it in firmly. If using a measuring cup, gently turn the bath bomb out onto parchment paper or wax paper and let dry overnight. Repeat with the remaining mixture. If using silicone molds, let the bath bombs dry overnight in the molds before popping them out.

6. Keep the bath bombs in a sealed bag or Mason jar, labeled and dated, to keep out moisture.

7. Use one bath bomb at a time. Drop it into the filled tub and watch your cares fizz away.

1 cup baking soda

½ cup citric acid

2 tablespoons coconut milk powder

2 tablespoons arrowroot powder, or cornstarch

1 tablespoon unrefined coconut oil, melted

20 drops coriander essential oil

20 drops lime peel essential oil

5 drops ylang-ylang essential oil

5 drops neroli essential oil

Witch hazel, in a small spray bottle

Swap it out: *If you don't have lime peel essential oil on hand, use another citrus essential oil such as lemon, sweet orange, or grapefruit.*

Bohemi Babe Herbal Mud Masks

ACNE, DRY SKIN, FINE LINES AND WRINKLES, SELF-ESTEEM • TOPICAL • **MAKES 8 TREATMENTS**

Safe for ages 5+

When you don't have time for a relaxing day at the spa, why not bring the spa home to you? This luxurious herbal clay mud mask is easy to mix up and chock-full of nutrients. It will help reduce fine lines and minimize pores. Roman chamomile essential oil is naturally anti-inflammatory and often used in facial care products to hydrate dry skin as well as reduce redness and irritation.

1. In a medium glass bowl, stir together the clay, oats, lavender buds, chamomile flowers, and flaxseed until combined.

2. Add the Roman chamomile and sweet orange essential oils.

3. Wearing gloves and using your hands, mix the essential oils into the powder until there are no clumps remaining.

4. Keep the mask in a sealed Mason jar, label and date your creation, and store in a cool, dark location for up to 2 years.

5. To use, mix 1 tablespoon of the dry mix with enough filtered water (or hydrosol, cooled herbal tea, or aloe vera juice) to create a paste.

6. Apply the herbal clay mask to your face, avoiding the hair, eyes, lips, and nostrils. Let the mask sit for 15 to 20 minutes. Mist your face with a facial toner if the mask gets too dry or itchy.

7. Rinse the mask from your face, then apply your favorite facial toner and moisturizer.

¼ cup white kaolin clay

1 tablespoon oats, finely ground

1 tablespoon dried lavender buds, finely ground

1 tablespoon dried chamomile flowers, finely ground

1 tablespoon ground flaxseed

10 drops Roman chamomile essential oil

15 drops sweet orange essential oil

Helpful hint: *Use a coffee grinder to grind the oats and herbs in this recipe. I find you can get a finer grind when they are combined and ground together.*

Detoxifying Charcoal Face Mask

ACNE, ECZEMA, SELF-ESTEEM • TOPICAL • **MAKES 8 TREATMENTS**

Safe for ages 5+

When stress and anxiety take over, the first place most people tend to show it is in their skin. Breakouts often occur during times of stress and anxiety. These breakouts can include acne, eczema, psoriasis, and even cold sores. When breakouts occur, this Detoxifying Charcoal Face Mask can help tame inflamed skin, reduce irritation, and draw out toxins. It is important to stay hydrated throughout the detox process—try drinking water infused with citrus fruits, fresh herbs, and cucumbers for a deluxe spa experience at home.

1. In a medium glass bowl, stir together the clay, charcoal, lavender buds, and tea leaves.

2. Add the lavender and grapefruit essential oils.

3. Wearing gloves and using your hands, mix the essential oils into the powder until there are no clumps remaining.

4. Keep the mask in a sealed Mason jar, label and date your creation, and store in a cool, dark location for up to 2 years.

5. To use, mix 1 tablespoon of the dry mix with enough filtered water (or hydrosol, cooled herbal tea, or aloe vera juice) to create a paste.

6. Apply the herbal clay mask to your face, avoiding the hair, eyes, lips, and nostrils. Let the mask sit for 15 to 20 minutes. Mist your face with a facial toner if the mask gets too dry or itchy.

7. Rinse the mask from your face, then apply your favorite facial toner and moisturizer.

¼ cup bentonite clay

2 tablespoons activated charcoal

1 tablespoon dried lavender buds, finely ground

1 tablespoon green tea leaves, finely ground

10 drops lavender essential oil

10 drops grapefruit essential oil

Swap it out: *If you don't have bentonite clay on hand, any type of clay will work in this recipe, including kaolin, rhassoul, or French green clay.*

Cooling Cucumber Chamomile Sheet Masks

DRY SKIN, FINE LINES AND WRINKLES, INFLAMMATION, STRESS •
AROMATIC, TOPICAL • **MAKES 1 TREATMENT**

Safe for all ages

Sheet masks first became popular in Korea and Japan but have since gained popularity all over the world for their unique ability to moisturize the skin. This recipe features Roman chamomile hydrosol, a byproduct of essential oil distillation that is great at hydrating dry, inflamed skin while also soothing frazzled nerves. Chamomile hydrosol is so gentle it does not need to be diluted like the essential oil. It's even safe to use on babies and small children.

¼ cup aloe vera gel

¼ cup Roman chamomile hydrosol

½ unpeeled cucumber, sliced

1 sheet mask

1. In a blender, combine the aloe vera gel, Roman chamomile hydrosol, and cucumber. Blend until the cucumber is completely puréed.

2. Place a fine-mesh sieve over a medium glass bowl and strain the mixture through it, pressing all the liquid through the strainer. Discard or compost the solids.

3. Wash your face and pat it dry.

4. Dip the dry sheet mask into the cucumber liquid, thoroughly soaking the mask. Let the sheet mask drip any excess liquids back into the bowl, but do not wring out the mask. Unfold the sheet mask and gently position it on your face.

5. Let the mask sit on your face for 30 minutes.

6. Peel the mask off and thoroughly rinse your face. You can then apply your favorite facial toner and moisturizer, if you wish. This mask can be used daily.

Helpful hint: *You can find pre-cut, dry cotton sheet masks on Amazon or other online beauty retailers. You can purchase a pack of 100 for about $5. If you made this mask recipe twice a week, 100 pre-cut masks would last you roughly a year. With a single sheet mask soaked in serum selling for upward of $10 each, that's a huge savings.*

Restore and Hydrate Facial Toner

DRY SKIN, FINE LINES AND WRINKLES, INSOMNIA, NERVOUS TENSION, OILY SKIN •
TOPICAL • **MAKES ABOUT 4 OUNCES**

Safe for all ages

Toning is one of the most neglected steps in facial cleansing. Toning helps remove excess oils and dead skin cells after washing. Toning also restores your face's pH, closes your pores, and helps moisturizer penetrate your skin better. This refreshing toner is great for all skin types, including dry, oily, or mature skin.

1. In a 4-ounce spray bottle, combine the witch hazel, aloe vera gel, vegetable glycerin, and lavender, frankincense, and neroli essential oils. Gently swirl the bottle to mix.

2. Add distilled water to fill the bottle. Cover the bottle.

3. To use, shake well and spray the toner onto a freshly cleansed face, avoiding contact with the eyes. Follow with a facial moisturizing oil.

4. Label and date your creation and store any unused spray in a cool, dark location for up to 1 year.

¼ cup witch hazel

1 tablespoon aloe vera gel

1 teaspoon vegetable glycerin

10 drops lavender essential oil

10 drops frankincense essential oil

6 drops neroli essential oil

Distilled water, to fill

Swap it out: *Boost the age-defying properties in this facial toner by substituting rose hydrosol for the filtered water. Gentle and healing, rose hydrosol is great for all skin types and will enhance the scent of this blend.*

Rapunzel's Deep Conditioning Hair Mask

ANXIETY, HEADACHES, THINNING HAIR • AROMATIC, TOPICAL • **MAKES 1 TREATMENT**

Safe for ages 4+

Stress and anxiety can sometimes lead to hair-related symptoms, including hair loss, balding, and slow growth. Although genetics also play a big role in these conditions, there are natural remedies that can help reduce these symptoms and improve your hair's luster, shine, and strength. The essential oil combination used here will not only promote healthy hair growth, but your scalp also doubles as a gentle diffuser, giving you a soothing aromatherapeutic experience while conditioning your hair and scalp.

1. In a small glass bowl, stir together the argan oil, avocado oil, and neroli, bergamot, and coriander essential oils.

2. Wet your hair. Apply the mixture to your damp hair, working from the ends to the roots. Massage the oil into your scalp to promote hair growth.

3. Leave the conditioning oil treatment on your hair for 1 to 2 hours before using shampoo.

4. Shampoo your hair twice before conditioning with your regular conditioner.

5. Repeat once a week to stimulate hair growth.

1 teaspoon argan oil

1 teaspoon avocado oil

2 drops neroli essential oil

2 drops bergamot essential oil

1 drop coriander essential oil

Awesome addition: *Rich in ricinoleic acid and omega-6 fatty acids, castor oil accelerates circulation at the hair's roots, helping to quickly strengthen and grow hair. Castor oil is also great at preventing hair breakage and reducing split ends. Add 1 teaspoon castor oil to this recipe for an even deeper conditioning treatment.*

Good Night, Sleep Tight Bath

HEADACHES, INSOMNIA, MUSCLE TENSION, NAUSEA, RESTLESS LEG SYNDROME, STRESS •
AROMATIC, TOPICAL • **MAKES 1 TREATMENT**

Safe for ages 4+

This bath was originally designed with my son in mind, but it worked so well the adults in the house began using it, too. Lavender and marjoram essential oils are great at relaxing muscles and calming the mind, and chamomile essential oil calms both the digestive system and the nervous system, making this sleepy time bath the perfect way to end the day. Pair this bath with a cup of chamomile and mint tea. Not only will the tea relax you for bedtime, but having a bedtime ritual like dimming the lights, enjoying a bath, and drinking a soothing cup of tea can help condition your brain for relaxation and sleep.

1. In a medium glass bowl, stir together the avocado oil and Roman chamomile, sweet marjoram, and lavender essential oils.

2. Using a spoon, stir the Epsom salt into the oil mixture.

3. Pour the mixture under the running water as you fill the bathtub.

4. Soak in the tub for at least 20 minutes for maximum benefits.

2 tablespoons avocado oil, or another liquid carrier oil

3 drops Roman chamomile essential oil

3 drops sweet marjoram essential oil

3 drops lavender essential oil

1 cup Epsom salt

Helpful hint: *Don't want to deal with a slippery tub after the bath? Substitute your favorite unscented shampoo or bubble bath for the avocado oil in this recipe.*

Energizing Grapefruit Coffee Body Scrub

CELLULITE, DEPRESSION, ENERGY, INFLAMMATION, MENTAL FATIGUE •
TOPICAL • **MAKES ABOUT 8 OUNCES**

Safe for ages 10+

Coffee is great for waking you up, but did you know the caffeine in coffee helps reduce cellulite? This rejuvenating sugar scrub will wake you up while it exfoliates, leaving behind soft, glowing skin. Grapefruit essential oil contains the anti-inflammatory enzyme bromelain, which also helps break down cellulite. With the combined powers of grapefruit and coffee, this body scrub will have you feeling energized and at your best.

1. In a medium glass bowl, stir together the sugar, coffee, coconut oil, and grapefruit essential oil.

2. Massage the scrub onto the skin. Rinse it off with warm water. (Caution: The tub or shower may be slippery after rinsing.)

3. Keep the scrub in a Mason jar, label and date your creation, and store in a cool, dry location for 6 to 9 months.

¾ cup sugar

¼ cup finely ground coffee beans

¼ cup to ½ cup unrefined coconut oil, or another liquid carrier oil, melted

30 drops grapefruit essential oil

Swap it out: *Out of sugar? Use salt instead.*

Every Day's Your Birthday Cake Sugar Body Scrub

ANXIETY, DEPRESSION, SELF-ESTEEM, STRESS • TOPICAL • **MAKES ABOUT 8 OUNCES**

Safe for ages 2+

Every once in a while we all need to be treated like we're special. I love to spend time celebrating myself with this sweet sugar scrub that makes me feel happy and celebrated. Vanilla essential oil is a wonderfully uplifting essential oil that can make you feel comfortable, safe, and content. Mix in your favorite naturally colored sprinkles and get the party started!

1. In a medium glass bowl, stir together the sugar, coconut oil, lemon zest, vanilla essential oil, and sprinkles as desired.

2. Massage the scrub onto the skin. Rinse with warm water. (Caution: The tub or shower may be slippery after rinsing.)

3. Keep your body scrub in a Mason jar, label and date your creation, and store in a cool, dry location for 6 to 9 months.

1 cup sugar

¼ cup unrefined coconut oil, melted

Grated zest of 1 lemon

20 drops vanilla essential oil

Naturally colored sprinkles, for mixing

Swap it out: *Replace the lemon zest in this recipe with grapefruit, lime, or orange zest to mix it up.*

Grapefruit Lavender Body Butter Bars

DEPRESSION, DRY SKIN, MENTAL FOCUS, NERVOUS TENSION, STRESS •
AROMATIC, TOPICAL • **MAKES ABOUT 6 OUNCES**

Safe for ages 2+

Body butter is the most luxurious way to moisturize your skin. These body butter bars are compact and great for travel. The sweet citrusy scent of grapefruit essential oil and the heady aroma of lavender will calm your mind and lift your spirits.

1. In a small pan over low heat, melt the coconut oil, shea butter, and beeswax. Remove the pan from the heat.

2. Add the grapefruit and lavender essential oils. Stir to combine.

3. Pour the mixture into molds (I have used mini muffin tins, though my favorite molds are silicone baking molds—not only do you get fun shapes for all types of seasons/themes, but they are easier to remove the bars from). For quick cooling, put the filled molds into the freezer for 20 minutes. Otherwise, let sit on the counter for 4 to 6 hours to harden.

4. Once cooled and hardened, remove from the molds and transfer to a glass Mason jar. Label and date your creation and store in a cool, dark location for up to 1 year.

5. To use, melt the bar in the palms of your hands and rub it all over your body for effective moisturizing with a delightful scent.

¼ **cup unrefined coconut oil**

2 **tablespoons shea butter**

¼ **cup beeswax**

60 **drops grapefruit essential oil**

30 **drops lavender essential oil**

Awesome addition: *For an extra luxurious body butter, replace 2 tablespoons of the coconut oil with 2 tablespoons mango butter. This will create the perfect combination of butter and oil, giving your skin a soft, supple feeling.*

Don't Worry Be Happy Lip Balm

ANXIETY, DEPRESSION, DRY OR CHAPPED LIPS, SEASONAL AFFECTIVE DISORDER •
TOPICAL • **MAKES ABOUT 3 OUNCES**

Safe for ages 4+

When the cold winter air chaps your lips and blows away the warm fuzzy feelings, this sweet lemon cookie–scented lip balm will be a ray of sunshine while softening and moisturizing your lips.

1. In a small pan over low heat, melt the coconut oil, beeswax, and mango butter. Remove the pan from the heat.

2. Stir in the castor oil and lemon, Roman chamomile, and vanilla essential oils.

3. Pour the melted lip balm mixture into lip balm tubes, ½-ounce metal tins, or recycled mint tins, and let it cool and harden. Label and date your creation.

4. Apply as needed to lips as a healing moisturizer.

Helpful hint: *Pour the lip balm into half of a cute locket and wear it around your neck.*

3 tablespoons unrefined coconut oil

1½ tablespoons beeswax

1 tablespoon mango butter

1 tablespoon castor oil

20 drops lemon essential oil

10 drops Roman chamomile essential oil

10 drops vanilla essential oil

Herban Spice Calming Beard Oil

ANXIETY, DRY HAIR, ITCHINESS, SELF-ESTEEM, STRESS •
AROMATIC, TOPICAL • **MAKES ABOUT 1 OUNCE**

Safe for ages 6+; not safe for pregnant or nursing women

Beard oil like this one helps condition, smooth, and straighten beards so they don't look scraggly. It also helps moisturize and soothe the skin underneath the beard, preventing itchiness. This essential oil blend smells divine with just the right balance of the earth, wood, spice, and citrus notes. The heady aroma diffuses off the beard, giving you a sense of calm throughout the day.

1. In a medium glass bowl, stir together the hemp seed oil, avocado oil, apricot kernel oil and bergamot, frankincense, cardamom, and Atlas cedarwood essential oils.

2. Pour the mixture into a 1-ounce dark glass bottle with a dropper top. Label and date your creation.

3. To use, after dampening your beard, drop 5 to 8 drops (depending on beard size) into your palm and massage the blend into your beard. Using your fingers, comb through your beard completely to distribute the oil evenly.

Helpful hint: *Dampen your beard slightly before applying any beard-care products. Hair has an aqueous layer that can prevent proper absorption, but when dampened with water-based ingredients, your hair absorbs the oils better. Although water will work just fine, I suggest spraying your beard with facial toner as the perfect pre-beard grooming ritual.*

1 tablespoon hemp seed oil

1½ teaspoons avocado oil

1½ teaspoons apricot kernel oil

10 drops bergamot essential oil

5 drops frankincense essential oil

3 drops cardamom essential oil

3 drops Atlas cedarwood essential oil

Earthen Faerie Solid Perfume

Safe for ages 2+

The subtle earthy notes of cedarwood combined with the sweet, floral aromas of neroli and lavender blend well with the herbaceous smell of marjoram. This intoxicating perfume can help increase mental focus, calm a nervous mind, and help you relax if feeling tightly wound.

1. In a double boiler set over medium heat, combine the grapeseed oil, coconut oil, and beeswax. Heat until the beeswax is melted. Remove the double boiler from the heat.

2. Add the sweet marjoram, lavender, Atlas cedarwood, and neroli essential oils and mix well until combined.

3. Pour the mixture into the containers you have chosen for your solid perfume. Label and date your creation.

4. To use, gently warm the top of the solid perfume with your finger and apply the perfume behind your ears, at the base of your neck, and to your wrists.

3 tablespoons grapeseed oil

1 tablespoon unrefined coconut oil

1 tablespoon beeswax pastilles

30 drops sweet marjoram essential oil

20 drops lavender essential oil

10 drops Atlas cedarwood essential oil

3 drops neroli essential oil

Helpful hint: *My favorite containers to store this solid perfume in are locket necklaces. They make cute gifts, look adorable, and even diffuse the scent from the locket as you wear it. Use a dropper to get the melted liquid into the lockets without making a mess.*

Paint and Sniff Aromatic Art

ANXIETY, DEPRESSION, OVERSTIMULATION, STRESS •
AROMATIC • **MAKES ENOUGH FOR 1 PAINTING**

Safe for ages 2+

We all know that Bob Ross was one happy dude, and when life gets overwhelming, I like to experiment with organoleptic art—art involving the use of your senses of smell, touch, and sight. It's taking the Bob Ross attitude to a whole new level. Individually, each of these scented paint colors smells soothing, but, as you begin to combine colors and express yourself on your canvas, you'll notice the scent transforms your work of art from an item of singular beauty into a complex masterpiece.

1. Pour roughly 1 tablespoon of each individual paint color into eight individual small bowls.

2. For each paint color, stir in the color-corresponding essential oil, mixing well to combine.

3. Paint with the aromatherapeutic paints individually at first, then continue by mixing and adding colors. Recognize how the aromas transform with the artwork. The art will still give off a scent for a few hours after drying.

Nontoxic acrylic paint, in a variety of colors, such as yellow, orange, purple, blue, etc. (you'll need 1 tablespoon of each color)

Various essential oils, corresponding to the following paint colors listed, or your choice (you'll need 25 drops of each oil)

Canvas

Paintbrushes

Blue tansy essential oil = blue paint

Cedarwood essential oil = brown paint

Frankincense essential oil = black paint

Grapefruit essential oil = red paint

Lavender essential oil = purple paint

Lemon essential oil = yellow paint

Roman chamomile essential oil = white paint

Sweet orange essential oil = orange paint

Multi-Sensory Stress Dough

ANXIETY, DEPRESSION, NERVOUS TENSION, OVERSTIMULATION, STRESS •
AROMATIC • **MAKES 5 DIFFERENT COLORS**

Safe for ages 2+

Just like the Paint and Sniff Aromatic Art (page 56), this Multi-Sensory Stress Dough is another form of organoleptic art—art involving the use of your senses of smell, touch, and sight. This playdough combines the calming movements of kneading dough with the uplifting aromatic scents of essential oils. Kneading this dough during times of high stress and anxiety can help reduce feelings of overstimulation, calm a panic attack, and relax a little one for naptime.

1. In a medium saucepan over medium heat, stir together the flour, salt, coconut oil, cream of tartar, and water. Heat the mixture, stirring constantly. The dough will begin to get lumpy. Continue stirring for 1 to 2 minutes more until the dough comes together in a ball.

2. Remove the dough from the pan and wrap it in plastic wrap to prevent it from drying out while it cools, about 30 minutes.

3. Unwrap the dough and divide it into 5 equal balls. Mix one color and its corresponding essential oil into each ball of dough, kneading them well to distribute the color and scent evenly.

4. Store the dough in a sealed container, labeled and dated, when not in use. This multi-sensory stress dough will keep for 1 year or longer, if properly stored.

1 cup all-purpose flour

½ cup salt

1½ tablespoons unrefined coconut oil

2 teaspoons cream of tartar

1 cup filtered water

Food coloring, to correspond to the following colors

Various essential oils, to correspond to the following list

Pink = 5 drops grapefruit essential oil

Purple = 5 drops lavender essential oil

Yellow = 5 drops chamomile essential oil

Orange = 5 drops bergamot essential oil

Green = 5 drops coriander essential oil

"No-Sew" Soothing Lavender Eye Pillow

ANXIETY, HEADACHES, INFLAMMATION, STRESS, TENSION •
AROMATIC, TOPICAL • **MAKES 1 TREATMENT**

Safe for ages 2+

Aromatherapy eye pillows have many benefits and uses for self-care. When cooled in the freezer they can relieve eye tension, headaches, puffy dark circles, and even fevers. When used after being warmed in the microwave, aromatherapy eye pillows can relieve headaches and soothe nervous tension. These "no-sew" eye pillows are extremely easy to make—even the kiddos can make their own.

1. In a medium glass bowl, mix the flaxseed and lavender buds until evenly combined.

2. Add the lavender essential oil and stir with a spoon to mix.

3. Pour the mixture into the sock and tie a knot at the open end.

4. To use hot, microwave the pillow for 15 to 30 seconds, or until it's warm but not too hot to the touch. Use the warm eye pillow for headaches, muscle pains, sprains, and strains. To use cold, put the eye pillow into a sealable bag to keep moisture from getting into the pillow and place it in the freezer overnight. Apply to the forehead or back of the neck when you are feeling overheated or ill. Lay the cold eye pillow over the eyes during meditation for added aromatherapeutic benefit.

1¼ cups flaxseed

¾ cup dried lavender buds

5 drops lavender essential oil

1 clean crew sock

Swap it out: *For a soothing kid-friendly alternative, chamomile flowers and Roman chamomile essential oil make an excellent alternative to the lavender buds and lavender essential oil in this recipe.*

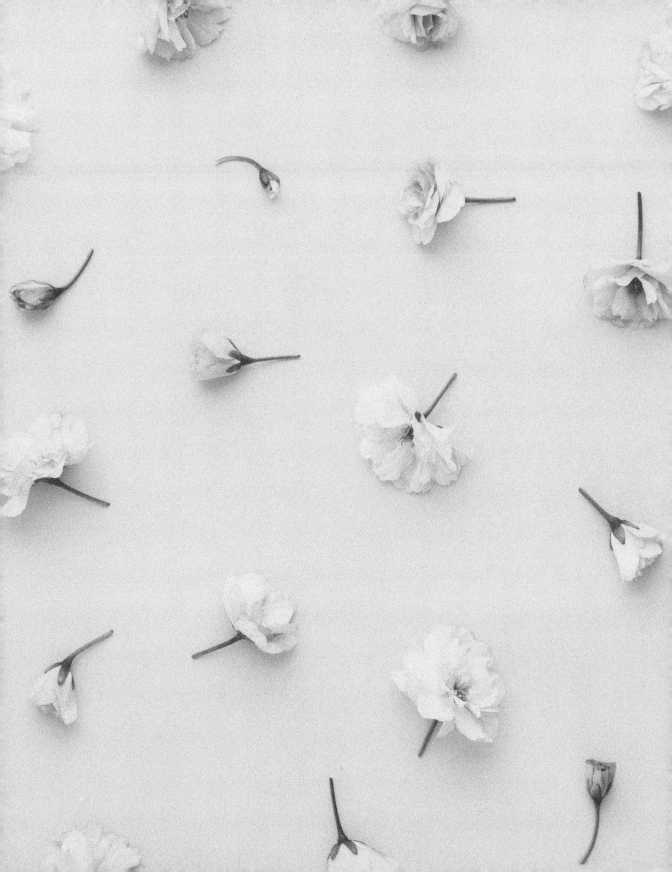

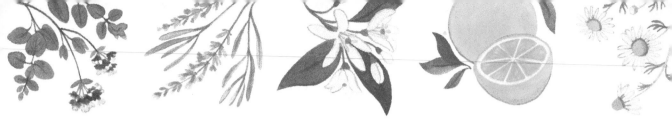

5

Breathe

Let the Sun Shine in Linen Spray

BRAIN FOG, DEPRESSION, ENERGY, MENTAL FOCUS • AROMATIC • **MAKES ABOUT 4 OUNCES**

Safe for ages 2+

When the sun's rays crawl over the horizon signifying a brand-new day, this sunshine-y linen spray will help bring the warm feeling of radiant light into your home. Spray your pillows, furniture, and curtains first thing in the morning and breathe in the fresh uplifting aromas as you perform the Bellows Breath Breathing Exercise (page 62) to start your day with sparkle and shine.

1. In a 4-ounce spray bottle, combine the witch hazel and lemon, bergamot, coriander, and lemongrass essential oils. Gently swirl the bottle to mix.

2. Add distilled water to fill the bottle.

3. Cover the bottle and shake well. Spray the mist into the air and on furniture and bedding (pillows, blankets, sheets, mattresses, and bedroom curtains).

4. Label and date your creation and store in a cool, dark location for up to 1 year.

¼ cup witch hazel

60 drops lemon essential oil

60 drops bergamot essential oil

30 drops coriander essential oil

15 drops lemongrass essential oil

Distilled water, to fill

Swap it out: *For an even sunnier aroma, substitute melissa hydrosol for the water in this recipe. Melissa hydrosol is an uplifting hydrosol that can help calm your nerves during times of high tension and worry. This fresh uplifting hydrosol has an earthy floral scent reminiscent of an herb garden after the rain.*

CONTINUED ▸

Bellows Breath Breathing Exercise

1. Sit up straight, extending your spine and relaxing your shoulders. Take a few deep breaths in and out through your nose. Every time you inhale, make sure your belly is expanding completely as you breathe.

2. Start bellows breathing by exhaling forcefully through your nose and inhaling forcefully through your nose. Each in-and-out breath should take one second.

3. Your breath should come from the diaphragm. Make sure your head, shoulders, neck, and chest are still while you take deep belly breaths in and out.

4. Breathe through a round of 10 bellows breaths for your first sequence, then take a break and breathe naturally for 15 to 30 seconds, observing the sensations in your mind and body.

5. Begin the next round. This time complete 20 bellows breaths, then take a break and breathe naturally for 30 seconds.

6. After the break, continue with a third, and final, round of 30 bellows breaths.

7. Always listen to your body during this practice. This is a safe practice, but beginners may feel light-headed or dizzy. If you feel light-headed or dizzy, pause for a few minutes and breathe regularly. When you feel up to it, try another round of bellows breathing, but take it easy.

Rainbows and Unicorns Perfume Oil

ANGER, GRIEF, SADNESS, STRESS • AROMATIC, TOPICAL • **MAKES ABOUT ⅓ OUNCE**

Safe for ages 6+

When it seems like reality is putting too much weight on your shoulders, take a moment to visit your imagination, where rainbows and unicorns are as prevalent as ice cream and cotton candy. Applying this sweet, uplifting blend and spending just 5 minutes performing the Alternate Nostril Breathing Exercise will lift the weight off your shoulders and put a smile on your face—even on the cloudiest of days.

1. In a ⅓-ounce glass roll-on bottle, combine the tangerine, neroli, and vanilla essential oils.

2. Add fractionated coconut oil to fill the bottle. Place the rollerball cap on the bottle and gently swirl the bottle to mix. Label and date your creation.

3. To use, roll the perfume onto the nape of your neck, behind your ears, and on your wrists. Gently massage it in.

6 drops tangerine essential oil

2 drops neroli essential oil

2 drops vanilla essential oil

Fractionated coconut oil, to fill

Swap it out: *Grapeseed oil is my favorite carrier oil to use in perfume oils because it is not greasy, it sinks into the skin quickly, and it carries the scent longer than other oils. For the longest-lasting scent, substitute grapeseed oil for the fractionated coconut oil in this recipe.*

Alternate Nostril Breathing Exercise

1. While practicing alternate nostril breathing, your breath should be slow, smooth, and continuous.

2. Find a quiet place and sit in a comfortable position. Cross your legs.

3. Place your thumb over your right nostril, closing it. Exhale fully through your left nostril.

4. Inhale through your left nostril.

5. Close the left nostril, open the right, and exhale through your right nostril.

6. Inhale through the right nostril and place your thumb over the right nostril.

7. Open the left nostril and exhale through the left nostril.

8. This is one complete cycle. Continue for up to 5 minutes.

9. Always end this exercise by exhaling through your left nostril.

Good Morning Beautiful Facial Moisturizer

DULL SKIN, FINE LINES AND WRINKLES, NEGATIVE THOUGHTS, SELF-ESTEEM •
AROMATIC, TOPICAL • **MAKES ABOUT 1 OUNCE**

Safe for ages 6+

This facial moisturizer will not only perk up dull, lackluster skin: It will also perk up your attitude for a bright, beautiful start to your day. This luxurious facial moisturizer will leave your skin soft and supple while erasing wrinkles and worry lines. When paired with the Beauty Breath Exercise, this blend will help ease nervousness and boost self-esteem.

1. In a 1-ounce pump-top bottle, combine the hemp seed oil, rosehip seed oil, argan oil and coriander, grapefruit, neroli, and basil essential oils. Gently swirl the bottle to mix. Label and date your creation.

2. After cleansing and toning your face, dispense 1 to 3 drops of moisturizing serum onto your palm, rub your hands together, and gently massage the serum onto your face. I recommend 1 drop of oil for your morning application and 2 or 3 drops of oil for your evening application.

1 tablespoon hemp seed oil

1½ teaspoons rosehip seed oil

1½ teaspoons argan oil

3 drops coriander essential oil

3 drops grapefruit essential oil

1 drop neroli essential oil

1 drop basil essential oil

Did you know? *Basil essential oil is well known for its ability to clear mental fog, boost cognitive function, and improve focus and concentration. It's the perfect essential oil to get your morning started beautifully!*

Beauty Breath Exercise

If pairing this exercise with the Good Morning Beautiful Facial Moisturizer, after rubbing the oil in the palm of your hands, massage the oil into your face while practicing this exercise.

1. Inhale for a count of 10.

2. Hold this breath for a count of 10.

3. Exhale for a count of 10.

4. Do this 10 times.

Cheer Up Buttercup Facial Steam

DEPRESSION, INSOMNIA, OVERSTIMULATION, TENSION • AROMATIC • **MAKES 1 TREATMENT**

Safe for ages 7+

Facial steams have been used for centuries, dating as far back as Cleopatra's era. They're not only beneficial for your pores, but they also provide another great method for inhaling the medicinal benefits of aromatic oils and herbs. This facial steam is designed to relax nervous tension, boost a sour mood, and clear negative energy. Pair this remedy with the Equal Breathing Exercise (page 66) to find your balance and achieve happiness.

1. Fill a medium glass bowl with boiling water. Add the geranium, Roman chamomile, blue tansy, and lavender essential oils.

2. Drape a large towel over your head and neck to create a tent effect and lean over the bowl—no closer than 10 inches from the hot water to prevent a burn.

3. Close your eyes and breathe in deeply for up to 2 minutes at a time. Repeat as needed.

4. Use the corresponding Equal Breathing Exercise with this facial steam for maximum benefits.

Boiling water, to fill

1 drop **geranium essential oil**

1 drop **Roman chamomile essential oil**

1 drop **blue tansy essential oil**

1 drop **lavender essential oil**

Awesome addition: *Herbs can boost the medicinal benefits of this facial steam. Some of my favorite herbs to add to facial steams include lavender buds, chamomile flowers, rose petals, rosemary sprigs, and lemon balm.*

Add ¼ cup dried herbs to the bowl and pour the boiling water over the herbs. Cover the bowl with a towel to keep the herbal steam in the bowl. Let the herbs steep in the water for 5 minutes before adding the essential oils.

CONTINUED ▸

Equal Breathing Exercise

1. Come into a comfortable sitting or standing position. This can be done while holding your head over the Cheer Up Buttercup Facial Steam bowl.

2. Close your eyes, relax your shoulders, and close your mouth so your lips gently touch each other.

3. Inhale slowly through your nose for a count of 3.

4. Exhale slowly through your nose for a count of 3. This is one cycle.

5. Continue even inhales and exhales counting your breath.

6. Increase the count by 1 with every cycle, up to a count of 10.

7. Begin to shorten the breath length by 1 each round until you reach 3 again.

Breathe Your Worries Away Diffuser Blend

ANXIETY, INSOMNIA, NERVOUS TENSION, PANIC, STRESS • AROMATIC • **MAKES ½ OUNCE**

Safe for ages 2+

This diffuser blend was created to help melt away tension and stress. When you can feel the worries of your day weighing upon your shoulders, add this essential oil blend to your diffuser and follow the instructions for the Worrywart Breathing Exercise.

1. In a dark glass dropper-top essential oil bottle, combine the lavender, Roman chamomile, marjoram, rosalina, and Virginia cedarwood essential oils. Gently swirl the bottle to mix. Label and date your creation.

2. Add 8 to 10 drops to a diffuser and diffuse throughout the room in 30-minute intervals (30 minutes on, 30 minutes off).

Helpful hint: *This essential oil blend can also be applied topically from an aromatherapy roll-on bottle or used as a massage oil if diluted following the Traditional Dilution Chart (page 10).*

1 teaspoon lavender essential oil

¾ teaspoon Roman chamomile essential oil

¾ teaspoon sweet marjoram essential oil

¼ teaspoon rosalina essential oil

¼ teaspoon Virginia cedarwood essential oil

Worrywart Breathing Exercise

1. Find a calm, comfortable place to sit. Relax your shoulders and neck. Take a slow, deep inhale through your nose. Make sure you're breathing into your belly: You should see your abdomen moving in and out.

2. Slowly exhale through your mouth. As you exhale, purse your lips and keep your jaw relaxed.

3. Continue for 3 minutes.

Stage Fright Aromatherapy Roll-On

NERVOUS TENSION, SELF-ESTEEM, STAGE FRIGHT, WRITER'S BLOCK •
AROMATIC, TOPICAL • **MAKES ABOUT ⅓ OUNCE**

Safe for ages 4+

Does fear stop you from trying new things? Fear is a common emotion that every one of us experiences, but it's how we push through the fear that makes us grow. Aromatherapy can help lift you up when you feel like shrinking. This aromatherapy blend has the perfect balance of spicy, minty, and sweet aromas to give you the boost you need to perform at your best. Pair this remedy with the Lion's Breath Breathing Exercise to calm your nerves before public speaking or a presentation at work.

1. In a ⅓-ounce glass roll-on bottle, combine the bergamot, spearmint, cinnamon, and vanilla essential oils.

2. Add fractionated coconut oil to fill the bottle. Place the rollerball cap on and gently swirl the bottle to mix. Label and date your creation.

3. To use, roll the blend onto the nape of your neck, behind your ears, and on your palms. Gently massage it in. Cup the palms of your hands over your nose and mouth and breathe in confidence-building scents.

5 drops bergamot essential oil

2 drops spearmint essential oil

2 drops cinnamon leaf essential oil

1 drop vanilla essential oil

Fractionated coconut oil, to fill

Swap it out: *Grapeseed oil is my favorite carrier oil to use in perfume oils because it is not greasy, sinks into the skin quickly, and carries the scent longer than other oils. For the longest-lasting scent, substitute grapeseed oil for the fractionated coconut oil in this recipe.*

Lion's Breath Exercise

1. Kneel so your buttocks are resting on your feet.

2. Place your hands on your knees. Straighten your arms and extend your fingers.

3. Breathe in through your nose.

4. Exhale forcefully through your mouth, making a "ha" sound with your exhalation. As you complete your exhalation, open your mouth wide and stick your tongue as far out as possible, toward your chin.

5. Inhale, returning your face to a neutral position.

6. Repeat this exercise 4 to 6 times.

Panic Stopper Aromatherapy Inhaler

HORMONAL FLUCTUATIONS, OVERSTIMULATION, PANIC, RACING THOUGHTS •
AROMATIC • **MAKES 1 TREATMENT**

Safe for ages 2+

When panic takes over the body, you might find yourself hyperventilating, sweating profusely, and/or shaking uncontrollably. This portable personal aromatherapy inhaler is the perfect size to carry in your pocket or bag and pull out whenever you start to feel the walls closing in. Combine this aromatherapy inhaler with the Navy SEAL's Box Breathing Exercise to regain control when you feel panic at your doorstep.

1. In a small glass bowl, combine the grapefruit, lavender, Roman chamomile, and clary sage essential oils.

2. Using tweezers, add the personal aromatherapy inhaler wick (the cotton pad) to the bowl and roll it around until it's soaked up all the essential oils.

3. Using tweezers, transfer the wick to the inhaler tube. Close the tube and label and date the inhaler.

4. Inhale, as needed.

10 drops grapefruit essential oil

3 drops lavender essential oil

3 drops Roman chamomile essential oil

3 drops clary sage essential oil

1 clean wick for personal aromatherapy inhaler

Swap it out: *Both coriander and rosalina essential oils have a similar linalool content to lavender essential oil, making them great substitutes when you want to change up this recipe.*

Navy SEAL's Box Breathing Exercise

1. Expel all the air from your lungs.

2. Keep your lungs empty for 4 seconds.

3. Inhale through your nose for 4 seconds.

4. Hold the air in your lungs for 4 seconds.

5. Exhale for a count of 4 seconds.

6. Repeat for 5 minutes, as needed.

Take a Chill Pillow Spray

ANXIETY, INSOMNIA, NERVOUS TENSION, STRESS • AROMATIC • **MAKES ABOUT 4 OUNCES**

Safe for ages 2+

I originally designed this recipe for my son when he was a toddler. All parents know that after 6 p.m. a craze comes over children that can be hard to tame before bedtime. I created this blend to help my little one calmly move through his bedtime routine and easily go to sleep at night. This blend ended up working so well that I began using it myself—with great success. If you are having trouble sleeping at night, spray this on your pillows, mattress, and in your bedroom before bedtime and do the 4-7-8 Breathing Exercise to gently lull yourself into a deep slumber.

1. In a 4-ounce spray bottle, combine the witch hazel and lavender, tangerine, Roman chamomile, and vanilla essential oils. Gently swirl the bottle to mix.

2. Add distilled water to fill the bottle.

3. Cover the bottle and shake well. Spray the mist into the air and on furniture and bedding (pillows, blankets, sheets, mattresses, and bedroom curtains).

4. Label and date your creation and store in a cool, dark location for up to 1 year.

¼ cup witch hazel

60 drops lavender essential oil

60 drops tangerine essential oil

30 drops Roman chamomile essential oil

15 drops vanilla essential oil

Distilled water, to fill

Swap it out: *For an even chiller vibe, substitute chamomile hydrosol for the water in this recipe. Chamomile hydrosol has a sweet floral scent reminiscent of fresh apples and it is a soothing hydrosol that can help calm your nerves and relax the body for bedtime.*

CONTINUED ▸

4-7-8 Breathing Exercise

1. Sit against a wall with your back straight.

2. Place the tip of your tongue against the top of your mouth, just behind your top front teeth. Do your best to keep it there.

3. With your mouth closed, inhale slowly through your nose.

4. With force, exhale fully through your mouth and making a whooshing sound with your breath. As you exhale, feel the air move around and past your tongue.

5. Close your mouth. Breathe slowly and quietly in through your nose for 4 seconds.

6. Hold your breath for 7 seconds.

7. Exhale completely through your mouth, making the whooshing sound for 8 seconds.

8. Inhale again and repeat for 4 rounds.

Seashore Shower Steamers

CLARITY, DEPRESSION, MENTAL FOG, STRESS • AROMATIC • **MAKES 6 TO 8 SHOWER STEAMERS**

Safe for ages 2+

When your body is fatigued and your brain is in a fog, you need a mental reset to nudge you back to reality. These shower steamers will clear the fog and perk you up so you can get through your day without stress weighing you down. Pair these shower steamers with the Oceanic Breathing Exercise and watch all your worries float away with the tide.

1. Wearing gloves and using your hands, in a medium glass bowl, combine the baking soda, citric acid, and cornstarch until no clumps remain.

2. Add the coriander, Atlas cedarwood, and frankincense essential oils to the mixture and, using your gloved hands, thoroughly mix them into the powders, breaking up small clumps.

3. Spray the mixture 2 or 3 times with witch hazel and continue to mix using your gloved hands until you can pack the mixture like a snowball without it crumbling. Repeat spraying the mixture if it is still too dry to hold together.

4. Pack the mixture into a ¼-cup measuring cup or silicone molds, pressing the mixture in firmly. If using a measuring cup, gently turn the steamer out onto parchment paper or wax paper to dry overnight. Repeat with the remaining mixture. If using silicone molds, let the steamers dry overnight in the molds before popping them out.

5. Keep the shower steamers in a sealed Mason jar, label and date your creation, and store in a cool, dark location.

6. To use, place one shower steamer at the end of the bathtub or shower, avoiding direct contact with the water. Let it slowly dissolve while you shower and breathe in the aromas.

1 cup baking soda

½ cup citric acid

1 tablespoon cornstarch, or arrowroot powder or any type of clay

½ teaspoon coriander essential oil

25 drops Atlas cedarwood essential oil

25 drops frankincense essential oil

Witch hazel, in a small spray bottle

Helpful hint: *If you get to the end of the batch of shower steamers and the scent has evaporated, add 5 drops of the essential oil blend used in the recipe to the tops of the shower steamers to refresh the scent before using.*

CONTINUED ▶

Oceanic Breathing Exercise

1. Sit tall with your shoulders relaxed away from your ears. Close your eyes. To prepare, focus on your breath without trying to control it.

2. Inhale and exhale through your mouth (not your nose).

3. Bring your focus to your throat. On your exhales, begin to tighten the back of your throat by slightly tightening the passage of air. Think of yourself fogging up a window. You should hear a soft hissing sound.

4. Once you are comfortable with the exhale, apply the same contraction of the throat on your inhale. You should, once again, hear a soft hissing sound. It should sound like the ocean.

5. Once you feel comfortable controlling your throat while inhaling and exhaling, close your mouth and breathe through your nose. Continue to apply the same throat constriction you used when your mouth was open.

6. Continue this practice for as long as needed. It is also helpful to use this breathing technique throughout your yoga practice.

Peaceful Yogi Yoga Mat Spray

DEPRESSION, ENERGY, MENTAL CLARITY, SELF-ESTEEM, STRESS •
AROMATIC, CLEANING, TOPICAL • **MAKES ABOUT 4 OUNCES**

Safe for ages 2+; not safe for pregnant or nursing women

Yoga is the perfect way to start the day with a clear head, ready for whatever may come your way. This fresh, energizing yoga mat spray is multi-purpose and can be used to set the mood before your practice and to clean your mat afterward. Spray your mat and the air around you before using the Namaste Ninja Breathing Exercise to achieve mental clarity and focus and receive an energizing dose of happiness.

1. In a 4-ounce spray bottle, combine the witch hazel and grapefruit, lemon, frankincense, and basil essential oils. Gently swirl the bottle to mix.

2. Add distilled water to fill the bottle.

3. Cover the bottle and label and date your creation.

4. To use, shake well. Spray the mat and yourself (avoiding your face) before beginning your yoga practice. Afterward, thoroughly spray the mat and pat it dry with a towel.

¼ cup witch hazel

20 drops grapefruit essential oil

20 drops lemon essential oil

10 drops frankincense essential oil

5 drops basil essential oil

Distilled water, to fill

Swap it out: *Tea tree essential oil is well known for its antibacterial properties, but yogis also like to use it in their practice to help detoxify and cleanse the soul. Substitute tea tree hydrosol for the water in this recipe to boost its antibacterial cleaning powers and rejuvenate your mind as you practice yoga.*

CONTINUED ▸

Namaste Ninja Breathing Exercise

1. Mentally scan your body and notice how it feels when you inhale and exhale normally. Make note of any tension in your body you didn't notice before.

2. Take a slow, deep breath, inhaling through your nose.

3. Pay attention to your belly and upper body expanding as you breathe in.

4. Exhale in whatever way is most comfortable for you.

5. Breathe in this manner for several minutes, focusing on the rise and fall of your belly.

6. Imagine your inhale washing over you like a gentle wave of bright light.

7. Imagine your exhale carrying negative energy and upsetting thoughts away from you.

8. If you get distracted, gently bring your attention back to your breath.

9. Continue this practice for up to 20 minutes daily.

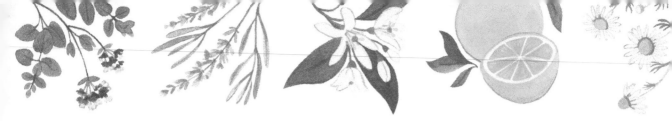

6

Meditate

Mindful Meditator Yoga Mat Spray

MENTAL FOCUS, MINDFULNESS, NERVOUSNESS, STRESS •
AROMATIC, CLEANING • **MAKES ABOUT 4 OUNCES**

Safe for ages 2+

Yoga and meditation go hand in hand. This yoga mat spray doubles as an aroma-therapeutic treatment to help you get into a meditative mind-set. This mindful meditator essential oil blend is especially good at clearing brain fog, relieving nervous tension, and soothing scattered thoughts so you can focus inward.

1. In a 4-ounce spray bottle, combine the witch hazel and lavender, bergamot, frankincense, Altas cedarwood, and sandalwood essential oils. Gently swirl the bottle to mix.

2. Add distilled water to fill the bottle.

3. Cover the bottle and label and date your creation.

4. To use, shake well. Spray the mat and yourself (avoiding your face) before beginning your yoga practice. Afterward, thoroughly spray the mat and pat it dry with a towel.

Swap it out: *Lavender is often used for its calming and soothing properties, but did you know it has antibacterial properties that rival tea tree essential oil? Substitute lavender hydrosol for the water in this recipe to boost its antibacterial cleaning powers and calm your mind for a deeper meditative practice.*

¼ cup witch hazel

20 drops lavender essential oil

20 drops bergamot essential oil

10 drops frankincense essential oil

5 drops Atlas cedarwood essential oil

5 drops sandalwood essential oil

Distilled water, to fill

CONTINUED ▶

Savasana Meditation

1. Begin by lying on your back, with your feet as wide as your mat. Let them flop open.

2. Relax your arms a few inches away from your body with palms facing the sky.

3. Tuck your chin in slightly toward your chest to lengthen the back of your neck.

4. Close your eyes and breathe normally. Notice the pace of your breath as you breathe in and out.

5. Mentally scan your body, starting with your toes and moving up.

6. Relax every muscle as you scan up your body, finally relaxing your jaw and scalp.

7. Lie on your mat with all your muscles relaxed, breathing in and out at a normal pace for at least 5 minutes, or until you feel you are done.

8. Don't immediately get up, but slowly bring awareness back into your body, first by gently wiggling your fingers and toes.

9. Finally, slowly roll on to your right side and gently raise up into a sitting position.

Sacred Smudge Diffuser Blend

EMOTIONAL UPHEAVAL, NEGATIVE THOUGHTS, STRESS, TENSION • AROMATIC • **MAKES 1 OUNCE**

Safe for ages 2+

When negative energy fills a space, it is an old tradition to cleanse the space by burning sage, also known as smudging. This essential oil blend is meant to cleanse *you* of negative thoughts, stress, and mood swings. The calming sweet scent will delight your senses and your soul.

1. In a dark glass dropper-top essential oil bottle, combine the clary sage, Roman chamomile, sweet marjoram, and lime essential oils. Gently swirl the bottle to mix. Label and date your creation.

2. Add 8 to 10 drops to a diffuser and diffuse throughout the room in 30-minute increments (30 minutes on, 30 minutes off).

1 teaspoon clary sage essential oil

¾ teaspoon Roman chamomile essential oil

¾ teaspoon sweet marjoram essential oil

½ teaspoon lime essential oil

Helpful hint: *This diffuser blend can be used topically when properly diluted. Simply mix 15 to 18 drops of this essential oil into 1 ounce of carrier oil, lotion, or butter.*

Sitting Meditation

1. Select a quiet time and place and begin by getting seated, erect, yet relaxed, on a cushion or chair.

2. Close your eyes and bring your full, present attention to whatever you feel around you and within you.

3. As you sit, feel the sensations of your body. Notice all the sounds and feelings, thoughts and expectations present. Allow them to come and go like the rise and fall of the ocean's waves. Be aware of these waves as they push and pull through your mind. Allow yourself to become more and more still with each fluid breath.

4. In the center of these waves, focus on your breath. Let the rhythm of your breathing be your focal point. Whenever you notice your thoughts straying and your attention being carried away, acknowledge it, then gently return your focus to your breath.

5. Continue this practice for 20 to 30 minutes. Open your eyes and look around you, taking in your reality, before getting up. Try to move through the rest of your day with this awareness, focusing on your breath when things get tough.

Dream Catcher Diffuser Blend

INSOMNIA, NIGHTMARES, STRESS, TENSION • AROMATIC • **MAKES 1 OUNCE**

Safe for ages 2+

When sleep eludes because of racing thoughts, stress, or bad dreams, this essential oil blend will help carry away your worries. Use this diffuser blend while you practice the Bedtime Meditation to clear your mind so you can fall into a peaceful and dreamy sleep.

1. In a dark glass dropper-top essential oil bottle, combine the lavender, Roman chamomile, sweet marjoram, neroli, and sweet orange essential oils. Gently swirl the bottle to mix. Label and date your creation.

2. Add 8 to 10 drops to a diffuser and diffuse throughout the room in 30-minute intervals (30 minutes on, 30 minutes off).

Helpful hint: *This diffuser blend can be used topically when properly diluted. Simply mix 15 to 18 drops into 1 ounce of carrier oil, lotion, or butter.*

1 teaspoon lavender essential oil

¾ teaspoon Roman chamomile essential oil

¾ teaspoon sweet marjoram essential oil

¼ teaspoon neroli essential oil

¼ teaspoon sweet orange essential oil

Bedtime Meditation

1. Start by setting the mood in your room. Make sure your bedroom is a comfortable temperature, your pillows are positioned where you like them, and any white noise or music needed is ready to go. Turn off the lights and get into bed.

2. Make yourself comfortable in bed, choosing whatever position feels the best for your body. Once you are comfortable, close your eyes and begin to focus on your breath, gently breathing in for a reverse count of 5 and breathing out for a reverse count of 5.

3. Continue this practice, focusing on the backward count of 5 with each inhale and exhale. Whenever your thoughts begin to stray from the count, gently bring your focus back to your breath and begin again.

Muse Journal Spray

ANXIETY, DEPRESSION, SELF-ESTEEM, STRESS • AROMATIC • **MAKES ABOUT 4 OUNCES**

Safe for ages 2+

Journaling is a wonderful way to sort out your thoughts and be mindful of the feelings you are experiencing. This journaling spray will help give you an aromatherapeutic edge by gently diffusing the scent off the pages as you work through your inner monologue. Pair this soothing spray with the Journal Reflection Meditation to calm your mind and unwind tension.

1. In a 4-ounce spray bottle, combine the witch hazel and bergamot, tangerine, Roman chamomile, and cinnamon essential oils. Gently swirl the bottle to mix.

2. Add distilled water to fill the bottle.

3. Cover the bottle and label and date your creation.

4. To use, shake well. Spray the mist onto the pages of an empty journal and let dry before writing in it. Store in a cool, dark location for up to 1 year.

¼ cup witch hazel

60 drops bergamot essential oil

60 drops tangerine essential oil

30 drops Roman chamomile essential oil

15 drops cinnamon leaf essential oil

Distilled water, to fill

Swap it out: *For a sweeter calming scent, substitute chamomile hydrosol for the water in this recipe. Chamomile hydrosol has a sweet floral scent reminiscent of fresh apples and is a soothing hydrosol that can help calm your nerves and relax the mind.*

Journal Reflection Meditation

Journaling is a great way to reflect on your feelings and get to know yourself better. As Eleanor Roosevelt once said, "Friendship with oneself is all-important, because without it one cannot be friends with anyone else in the world." Meditation through introspection journaling is easy. Simply sit for 20 minutes a day with your journal and write down your feelings, emotions, problems, and wins. One of the best ways to go deep within yourself is to use writing prompts and write what immediately comes to mind. Here are seven journal reflection writing prompts to get you started:

1. **Describe yourself, from a loved one's perspective.** It can be hard to imagine what others see when they look at you, but let's pretend for a moment that you are one of

CONTINUED ▸

your loved ones. Describe your best qualities, your favorite quirks, and the things that stand out about you from that person's perspective.

2. **Embark on the adventure of your lifetime.** Where would you go if there were no limitations? Tell this story like you just came home from this adventure and be sure to describe the feelings you felt throughout your adventure. Feelings are more important than physical descriptions of the beauty you see visually.

3. **Go beyond your comfort zone.** What scares you? Is it public speaking? Writing an original song and playing it in front of other people? Writing a short story for a contest? Write about three activities that put you outside your comfort zone and make a promise to start one of them in the next 7 days.

4. **What makes you want to dance when no one is looking?** Everyone has an "I am so excited I need to celebrate" dance. Whether it's because we're getting what we asked for, the universe is bringing us unexpected surprises, or we conquered a fear, we all like to celebrate when good things come to us. What would give you a reason to dance right now?

5. **Can a painful experience be a point of gratitude?** Pain is a natural part of life. In fact, all the best things that have come to you wouldn't have happened without a previous painful experience or moment. Sometimes it can be too difficult to see the positive while we are experiencing pain, but, after, we can look back and realize just how far we have come because of all our experiences. What is one painful past experience that was a catalyst for something good in your life?

6. **What are you passionate about?** If you were given a large sum of money to fuel your passion in whatever way you see fit, what would you do with it? Would you run a charity? Would you start a business? Would you travel the world and explore every crack and corner? Describe what you would do to follow your passions. What can you do to start working on your passions now, if you were to start small?

7. **Learn from your mistakes.** So, you made a mistake. Guess what? So did I! So has everyone else in this world. Literally everyone. Don't beat yourself up over it. Mistakes are merely lessons you need to learn—without them, you would have no growth. What mistakes have you made recently that you can forgive? What lessons did you learn from them?

Tropical Paradise Shower Steamers

ANXIETY, DEPRESSION, MENTAL FATIGUE, MOOD SWINGS •
AROMATIC • **MAKES 6 TO 8 SHOWER STEAMERS**

Safe for ages 2+

When that negative self-talk gets to be too much, it might be time to escape to paradise to renew your mind, body, and soul. The tropical scents of grapefruit, lime, and ylang-ylang combine to form a floral citrus scent that will carry away your worries with the water. Pair one of these shower steamers with the Waterfall Meditation to transport your senses to your own tropical paradise.

1. Wearing gloves and using your hands, in a medium glass bowl, combine the baking soda, citric acid, and cornstarch until there are no clumps remaining.

2. Add the grapefruit, lime, and ylang-ylang essential oils to the mixture and, using your gloved hands, thoroughly mix them into the powders, breaking up small clumps.

3. Spray the mixture 2 or 3 times with witch hazel and continue to mix, using your gloved hands, until you can pack the mixture like a snowball without it crumbling. Repeat spraying the mixture if it is still too dry to hold together.

4. Pack the mixture into a ¼-cup measuring cup or silicone molds, making sure to press the mixture in firmly. If using a measuring cup, gently turn the steamer out onto parchment paper or wax paper to dry overnight. Repeat with the remaining mixture. If using silicone molds, let the steamers dry overnight in the molds before popping them out.

5. Keep the shower steamers in a sealed Mason jar, label and date your creation, and store in a cool, dark location.

6. To use, place one shower steamer at the end of the bathtub or shower, avoiding direct contact with the water. Let it slowly dissolve while you shower, breathing in the steamy aromas.

1 cup baking soda

½ cup citric acid

1 tablespoon cornstarch, or arrowroot powder or any type of clay

½ teaspoon grapefruit essential oil

¼ teaspoon lime essential oil

¼ teaspoon ylang-ylang essential oil

Witch hazel, in a small spray bottle

Helpful hint: *If you get to the end of the batch of shower steamers and the scent has evaporated, add 5 drops of the essential oil blend used in the recipe to the tops of the shower steamers to refresh the scent before using.*

CONTINUED ▸

Waterfall Meditation

1. Stand facing the showerhead with your eyes closed and allow the water to run directly down the back of your neck.

2. As the water flows down your neck, become aware of the sensations around you. Focus on the feel of the water as it runs down your body. Focus on the sound of the water as each droplet converges. Allow your mind to quiet as you focus on the sound and sensations of the water.

3. Breathing steadily, in through your nose and out through your mouth, spend 5 minutes being present and aware of the water washing away any negative energy. As you inhale, imagine you are breathing in light and love. As you exhale, imagine you are breathing out all darkness and negativity.

Instant Gratification Aromatherapy Inhaler

ANXIETY, DEPRESSION, PANIC, STRESS • **AROMATIC** • **MAKES 1 TREATMENT**

Safe for ages 2+

It's common to feel like there is not enough time in the day to fit in space for personal reflection, but you only need 5 minutes a day to see the benefits of meditation. Whether it's right before you go into work, during your lunch break, or a quick breather between errands, this aromatherapy inhaler paired with the 5-Minute On-the-Go Mantra Meditation can help reduce anxiety, relieve panic, and mentally prepare you for the rest of your day.

1. In a small glass bowl, combine the grapefruit, sweet orange, lemon, and coriander essential oils.

2. Using tweezers, add the personal aromatherapy inhaler wick (the cotton pad) to the bowl and roll it around until it's soaked up all the essential oils.

3. Using tweezers, transfer the wick to the inhaler tube. Close the tube and label and date the inhaler.

4. Inhale, as needed.

10 drops grapefruit essential oil

3 drops sweet orange essential oil

3 drops lemon essential oil

3 drops coriander essential oil

1 clean wick for personal aromatherapy inhaler

Swap it out: *If you don't have coriander essential oil on hand, rosalina essential oil is a great substitute in this recipe. Rosalina is refreshing, like eucalyptus essential oil, but doesn't contain any cineole 1,8, making it safe for use around small children.*

CONTINUED ▸

5-Minute On-the-Go Mantra Meditation

Find a quiet private place where you can sit comfortably for this meditation. This can be done in your office, car, or even an empty conference room.

1. Set a timer with a gentle alarm for 5 minutes. Pick a simple mantra to repeat throughout the meditation. Some examples include:

   * Relax.
   * I am here. I am present. I am ready.
   * Be a warrior, not a worrier.
   * Don't let yesterday take up too much of today.
   * Anxiety is contagious, and so is calm.

2. Close your eyes and start by clearing your mind and focusing on your breath.

3. As you naturally inhale and exhale, repeat your chosen mantra in your mind until the timer goes off. Open your eyes and repeat your mantra one last time while taking in your surroundings.

Take a Walk Aromatherapy Roll-On

ENERGY, HEADACHES, PROCRASTINATION, TENSION • AROMATIC, TOPICAL • **MAKES 1 TREATMENT**

Safe for ages 6+

Sometimes sitting still isn't the answer to pent-up energy, frustration, and tension. A breath of fresh air and a healthy dose of nature can help unwind the knots that tension can tie. This refreshing blend is designed to relieve tension, reduce inflammation, and breathe energy back into your body. When paired with the Walking Meditation, you might find yourself feeling refreshed and ready to tackle the rest of your day.

1. In a ⅓-ounce glass roll-on bottle, combine the lavender, peppermint, and sweet marjoram essential oils.

2. Add fractionated coconut oil to fill the bottle. Place the rollerball cap on and gently swirl the bottle to mix. Label and date your creation.

3. To use, roll the blend onto the nape of your neck, behind your ears, and on your wrists. Gently massage it in.

Helpful hint: *This aromatherapy roll-on has multiple uses and is great at reducing the pain of tension headaches. Roll it onto your temples and rub in to ease the pain of a headache.*

6 drops lavender essential oil

4 drops peppermint essential oil

2 drops sweet marjoram essential oil

Fractionated coconut oil, to fill

CONTINUED ▶

Walking Meditation

1. Begin by walking at a naturally slow pace.

2. Relax, but maintain good posture. Your hands can be at your sides as you walk.

3. Breathing naturally, start to match your breath with your steps. Pay attention to how many steps you take for each inhale and each exhale. It is natural for the inhale to be slightly shorter than the exhale, so you may take 3 steps on your inhale and 4 steps on your exhale; that is okay.

4. In your mind, begin to consciously count your steps for each inhale and exhale. It might sound like this: 1-2-3, 1-2-3-4, 1-2-3, 1-2-3-4, or left-right-left, right-left-right-left, right-left-right, left-right-left-right, or inhale, exhale, inhale, exhale.

5. As you count your steps, be mindful and fully present. Though you are counting your steps, your mind may sometimes stray from this focus. When you realize you have strayed from your step count, acknowledge whatever arises and gently bring your thoughts back to your breath and start your count again.

Hug a Tree Jewelry Diffuser Blend

ANXIETY, MENTAL FOCUS, MENTAL FOG, NERVOUS TENSION • AROMATIC • **MAKES 1 OUNCE**

Safe for ages 2+

It is said that hugging a tree can ground you and bring you closer to Earth's soothing vibrational frequency. This essential oil blend is meant to honor the calm that breathing in the natural forest air can have on the human body. When the urban environment becomes too overstimulating, pair this blend with the Tree of Life Meditation and experience the warm embrace of Mother Nature.

1. In a dark glass dropper-top essential oil bottle, combine the lavender, fir needle, sweet marjoram, coriander, and Virginia cedarwood essential oils. Gently swirl the bottle to mix. Label and date your creation.

2. Add 3 to 5 drops of the essential oil blend to a jewelry diffuser and wear your jewelry to diffuse the scent around you.

Helpful hint: *This essential oil blend can also be used in your electric diffuser. Add 8 to 10 drops to the diffuser and diffuse throughout the room in 30-minute intervals (30 minutes on, 30 minutes off).*

1 teaspoon lavender essential oil

¾ teaspoon fir needle essential oil

¾ teaspoon sweet marjoram essential oil

¼ teaspoon coriander essential oil

¼ teaspoon Virginia cedarwood essential oil

CONTINUED ▸

Tree of Life Meditation

1. Begin by sitting on the ground, under a tree, in a comfortable position. If you have back problems use a chair, but for best results, you want your body to connect with the ground.

2. Sit straight, without slouching, but allow your spine to conform to its natural curve. Breathe slowly and deeply, quieting your mind, for 2 to 3 minutes.

3. Once you feel relaxed and focused, bring your attention to the base of your spine, or your root.

4. Imagine that each breath stretches your roots down into the earth. With each breath, feel these roots go through the ground, deep into the rich, dark soil that blankets our planet. Feel the coolness of the earth on your roots, as you dive deeper, away from air and light. Soon you will reach the end of Earth's hard crust. A space will open for your roots to continue deeper, toward the heart of our planet.

5. As your roots move into Earth's mantle, keep breathing steadily and stay focused. You may start to feel the heat emanating from Earth's outer core, as you move in closer to the molten center.

6. As you breathe, allow your roots to penetrate to the very center of the core, the heart of Earth. Sit here for a moment and bathe in your deep connection to Earth. Notice how grounded and centered you feel. Appreciate your body and the body of our Mother Earth. Thank her for all she provides for us.

7. Once you are ready, start pulling energy from the heart of Earth into your roots. With every breath, you pull up energy, power, grounding, and love. Watch as this energy rises through Earth's layers with each breath. Allow it to go up from the base of your spine, through your abdomen, your heart, your throat, and finally up through to the crown of your head.

8. Imagine this energy, light, and love burst through like the branches of a tree. Feel these branches reach up and out toward the sky. Sit here in this moment and bathe in your connection with Earth and sky.

9. When you feel ready, take a couple deep breaths and open your eyes.

Open Your Heart Aromatherapy Roll-On

ANGER, DEPRESSION, GRIEF, INSOMNIA • AROMATIC, TOPICAL • **MAKES 1 TREATMENT**

Safe for ages 2+

Oftentimes the stress and pain that can accompany anxiety cause us to protect ourselves by closing our hearts to love and light. This soothing floral-scented roll-on combines the relaxing properties of lavender with the sweet aromas of neroli and rose to calm the mind and soothe the body. When things seem bleak, pair this roll-on with the Loving Kindness Meditation to open your heart and feel the love.

6 drops lavender essential oil

4 drops rose essential oil

2 drops neroli essential oil

Fractionated coconut oil, to fill

1. In a ⅓-ounce glass roll-on bottle, combine the lavender, rose, and neroli essential oils.

2. Add fractionated coconut oil to fill the bottle. Place the rollerball cap on and gently swirl the bottle to mix. Label and date your creation.

3. To use, roll the blend onto the nape of your neck, behind your ears, and on your wrists. Gently massage it in.

Swap it out: *Steam-distilled rose essential oil can be very expensive because it requires large quantities of the flower to create a small amount of essential oil. Rose absolute is much cheaper to acquire and can be used in place of rose essential oil in this recipe.*

CONTINUED ▸

Loving Kindness Meditation

This meditation uses words, images, and feelings to evoke love and kindness toward yourself and others. With each repetition of the phrases in this meditation, you are putting intentions out into the universe and changing pathways in your brain.

1. Begin by sitting comfortably in a quiet space and clearing your mind. Relax your body and let go of any plans or preoccupations.

2. Gently breathe in and out and let your heart be soft. We start with loving ourselves before we can send love to others.

3. Inwardly, recite these phrases keeping a mental picture of yourself in the forefront of your mind and heart:

    ✳ May I be filled with loving kindness.
    ✳ May I be well in body, mind, and spirit.
    ✳ May I be calm and happy.

4. Repeat these phrases, letting the love wash over your mind and body. Continue this practice of meditating on loving kindness for yourself and watch as it grows.

5. Once you have developed a stronger sense of self-love, you can expand your meditation to include others. Instead of picturing yourself in your mind, picture your loved one and recite these phrases:

    ✳ May you be filled with loving kindness.
    ✳ May you be safe from inner and outer dangers.
    ✳ May you be well in body, mind, and spirit.
    ✳ May you be calm and happy.

Light Up Your Life Aromatherapy Candles

ANXIETY, MENTAL FOCUS, MENTAL FOG, OBSESSIVE BEHAVIORS • AROMATIC • **MAKES 1 CANDLE**

Safe for ages 2+

There is something soothing about a candlelit room filled with the sweet earthy aromas of herbs, flowers, and trees. Candles, with their dancing flames, have the ability to entrance those who watch them and to cast a warm light into dark places. Use these candles as a part of your normal meditation routine or try using them with the Flame Gaze Meditation.

1. In a medium glass measuring cup, melt the soy wax flakes in the microwave on high power, stirring every 30 seconds.

2. Once melted, stir in the coriander, sweet marjoram, Roman chamomile, and Atlas cedarwood essential oils. Pour the scented wax into a clean recycled candle jar.

3. Add the wick, centering it in the middle of the jar.

4. Leave the candle to cool and harden. Trim the wick with scissors before lighting for the first time.

Swap it out: *Although soy wax is my preferred wax for candle making, you can also make candles with all types of wax, including beeswax, carnauba wax, and candelilla wax. If you don't have soy wax on hand, use any wax you have available.*

2 cups soy wax flakes

30 drops coriander essential oil

30 drops sweet marjoram essential oil

30 drops Roman chamomile essential oil

10 drops Atlas cedarwood essential oil

1 recycled candle jar, or Mason jar

1 candlewick

CONTINUED ▸

Flame Gaze Meditation

1. Set up your lighted candle at eye level to prevent neck or back strain. Dim the lights in the room and come to a comfortable seated position, about 3 to 6 feet away from the flame so your gaze naturally falls on it.

2. Take a few long, deep breaths, relaxing your body, and bring your focus to the candle flame. Soften your gaze and become enthralled with the flame as it dances its hypnotic dance.

3. As you stare at the flickering flame, your mind may wander through its usual paths of thought. Accept those thoughts and gently refocus your concentration and awareness on the flame.

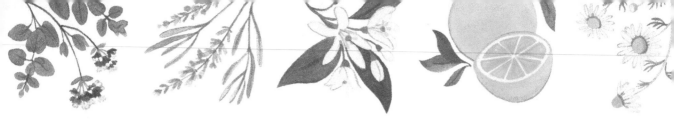

7

Restore

Sweet Dreams Magnesium Massage Spray

INSOMNIA, MUSCLE PAIN, RESTLESS LEG SYNDROME, RESTLESS MIND, TENSION •
TOPICAL • **MAKES ABOUT 4 OUNCES**

Safe for ages 2+ (use half the amount of essential oils for children 2 to 4 years of age)

Magnesium deficiency is extremely common and can cause various symptoms, including migraines, anxiety, mood swings, insomnia, and muscle spasms. This bedtime spray combines the power of relaxing essential oils and magnesium to help calm and soothe your mind and body for sleep.

1. In a 4-ounce spray bottle, combine the fractionated coconut oil, vegetable glycerin, and the lavender, sweet orange, sweet marjoram, and Atlas cedarwood essential oils. Gently swirl the bottle to mix.

2. Add magnesium oil to fill the bottle.

3. Cover the bottle and label and date your creation.

4. Shake well before use.

Note: *If you are new to using a magnesium spray, your skin may begin to itch at first. If that occurs, dilute the recipe with 2 tablespoons distilled water before adding the magnesium oil. You can use the recipe at regular strength when it's time to refill your bottle.*

Helpful hint: *You can use store-bought magnesium oil or easily make it yourself. To make your own magnesium oil, mix ½ cup magnesium flakes (magnesium chloride, not Epsom salt) with 3 tablespoons boiling water and stir until completely dissolved.*

1 tablespoon fractionated coconut oil

1 teaspoon vegetable glycerin

30 drops lavender essential oil

20 drops sweet orange essential oil

10 drops sweet marjoram essential oil

5 drops Atlas cedarwood essential oil

Magnesium oil, to fill

Magnesium Oil Bedtime Massage

Do this before bed.

1. Shake the Sweet Dreams Magnesium Massage Spray well before use and spray it onto your arms, legs, and feet.

2. Using a circular motion, gently massage the magnesium oil into your skin.

Sleep Deep Massage Oil

INSOMNIA, RACING THOUGHTS, REPETITIVE WAKEFULNESS, RESTLESS LEG SYNDROME •
TOPICAL • **MAKES ABOUT 2 OUNCES**

Safe for ages 2+ (use half the amount of essential oils for children 2 to 4 years of age)

Stress and anxiety can manifest as many symptoms in the body, but sleep issues are one of the worst symptoms to deal with. Without sleep your body goes into deeper states of distress: It becomes a vicious cycle of being stressed out and unable to sleep. Use this massage oil and treat yourself to the Bubbling Spring Bedtime Massage to relax before bedtime and get the sleep you need.

1. In a medium glass bowl, stir together the carrier oil and lavender, coriander, sweet marjoram, and bergamot essential oils.

2. Pour the mixture into a lotion pump bottle (or other preferred container). Label and date your creation and store in a cool, dark location.

¼ cup carrier oil of choice

15 drops lavender essential oil

10 drops coriander essential oil

10 drops sweet marjoram essential oil

5 drops bergamot essential oil

Swap it out: *For a small percentage of the population, lavender can have the opposite effect at bedtime. If this applies to you, substitute Roman chamomile essential oil for the lavender in this recipe.*

Bubbling Spring Bedtime Massage

The "bubbling spring" point is located on the sole of your foot. Look for a small depression on the ball of your foot that appears just above the middle of your foot when curling your toes.

1. Lie on your back with your knees bent into your chest so you can reach your feet with your hands.

2. With one foot in your hand, curl your toes and feel for the bubbling spring point. Using the Sleep Deep Massage Oil, apply firm pressure and, using a circular motion, massage the oil in. Repeat this process with the other foot.

Relax Your Back Tension Relief Massage Oil

HEADACHES, MUSCLE ACHES, STRESS, TENSION • TOPICAL • **MAKES ABOUT 2 OUNCES**

Safe for ages 6+; not safe for pregnant or nursing women

Some of the most common places to hold tension and stress are the lower back, neck, and shoulders. This spicy scented massage oil is designed to reduce inflammation and increase circulation by providing warmth to the area of concern.

1. In a medium glass bowl, stir together the carrier oil and sweet marjoram, peppermint, cinnamon, and black pepper essential oils.

2. Pour the mixture into a lotion pump bottle (or other preferred container). Label and date your creation and store in a cool, dark location.

Swap it out: *Peppermint essential oil has a high menthol content and, therefore, its use should be avoided around small children and pregnant or nursing women. To make this blend for children or pregnant women, substitute fir needle essential oil for the peppermint essential oil in this recipe.*

- ¼ **cup carrier oil of choice**
- **15 drops sweet marjoram essential oil**
- **10 drops peppermint essential oil**
- **10 drops cinnamon leaf essential oil**
- **5 drops black pepper essential oil**

Tension Relief Massage

Before performing this massage technique, first apply the Relax Your Back Tension Relief Massage Oil to your neck, shoulders, and lower back.

1. Lay out a yoga mat or towel. Bring two tennis balls with you to your yoga mat and lie face-up on the mat. Place the tennis balls under the middle of your back, one on each side of your spine.

2. Bend your knees, placing your feet firmly on the floor. Slowly move yourself back and forth so the tennis balls roll along your lower back.

3. To increase or decrease pressure from the tennis balls, use your legs to move your body horizontally up or down onto the balls.

Digestive Upset Massage Oil

CONSTIPATION, GAS, NAUSEA, UPSET STOMACH • TOPICAL • **MAKES ABOUT 2 OUNCES**

Safe for ages 2+ (use half the amount of essential oils for children 2 to 4 years of age)

When your stomach is topsy-turvy, essential oils can help relieve gas, indigestion, constipation, and even nausea. Although many consider peppermint essential oil to be the king of digestion help, it's not safe to use around babies and pregnant women; this remedy was designed with all users in mind. Ginger, coriander, and chamomile are all well known for their ability to calm and soothe any type of digestive upset.

1. In a medium glass bowl, stir together the carrier oil and sweet orange, Roman chamomile, coriander, and ginger essential oils.

2. Pour the mixture into a lotion pump bottle (or other preferred container). Label and date your creation and store in a cool, dark location.

Helpful hint: *If you are feeling queasy, you don't have to apply this oil to feel its benefits. Simply inhale directly from the bottle to ease a nauseated tummy.*

¼ cup carrier oil of choice

15 drops sweet orange essential oil

10 drops Roman chamomile essential oil

10 drops coriander essential oil

5 drops ginger essential oil

Digestive Abdominal Massage

1. Apply Digestive Upset Massage Oil directly to your abdomen.

2. In a clockwise manner, gently massage the oil into your abdomen.

Facial Massage Oil

FINE LINES AND WRINKLES, HEADACHES, STRESS, TENSION • TOPICAL • **MAKES ABOUT 1 OUNCE**

Safe for ages 2+

Facial massages increase circulation to your facial tissue, reducing the appearance of wrinkles and fine lines. This facial massage oil has a dual purpose: When combined with a facial massage, this can help reduce stress and promote a sense of calm, and when massaged into the forehead or temples it can help relieve a headache.

1. In a 1-ounce pump-top bottle, combine the hemp seed oil, grapeseed oil, pumpkin seed oil, and frankincense, Roman chamomile, and rose essential oils. Cover the bottle and gently swirl the bottle to mix. Label and date your creation. Store in a cool, dark location for up to 1 year.

- **1 teaspoon hemp seed oil**
- **½ teaspoon grapeseed oil**
- **½ teaspoon pumpkin seed oil**
- **3 drops frankincense essential oil**
- **2 drops Roman chamomile essential oil**
- **1 drop rose essential oil**

Swap it out: *Hemp seed oil is a must-have in any facial oil that I blend, but if you don't have the grapeseed and pumpkin seed oils on hand, use more hemp seed oil in their place, or elevate this recipe by using argan and rosehip seed oils.*

Facial Massage

1. Start with a freshly washed face. Apply a light layer of the facial massage oil.

2. Using the tips of your fingers, gently massage your lymph areas under your ears on the sides of your neck in a circular motion for 1 minute.

3. Using the same circular motions, move up to the sides of your face and gently massage your jaw, past the corners of your mouth, and up your cheekbones. Always push skin up (never down) to prevent sagging. Continue this for 1 minute.

4. Move to your forehead. Using broad circular motions, massage both sides simultaneously. Continue this for 1 minute.

5. Finally, position your fingertips at the outer edge of both eyebrows. Very gently massage them, working your way down under your eyes and up over the lids, making a circle over each eye. Continue this for 1 final minute.

Muscle Mender Massage Oil

HEADACHES, MUSCLE ACHES, STRESS, TENSION • TOPICAL • MAKES ABOUT 2 OUNCES

Safe for ages 6+; not safe for pregnant or nursing women

Exercise can be a great way to help manage stress and anxiety, but it can also result in sore muscles. When you are feeling muscle strain or pain from exercise—or extra-long hours on your feet—perform the Finish Line Leg Massage with this massage oil, which will gently warm and cool the targeted area, giving you sensations of ice and heat to reduce pain.

1. In a medium glass bowl, stir together the olive oil and lavender, sweet marjoram, peppermint, and cinnamon essential oils.

2. Pour the mixture into a lotion pump bottle (or other preferred container). Label and date your creation and store in a cool, dark location.

¼ cup olive oil

15 drops lavender essential oil

10 drops sweet marjoram essential oil

10 drops peppermint essential oil

5 drops cinnamon leaf essential oil

Swap it out: *Peppermint essential oil has a high menthol content and, therefore, its use should be avoided around small children and pregnant or nursing women. To make this blend for children or pregnant women, substitute rosalina essential oil for the peppermint essential oil in this recipe.*

Finish Line Leg Massage

Perform this massage for 10 minutes, after a run or workout session. Use the Muscle Mender Massage Oil to lubricate the massage, reduce inflammation, and soothe pain.

1. Using the massage oil, with your open hand and fingers relaxed, glide it over your legs starting with your feet and working your way up to your thighs. Stroke each leg 10 times, varying the intensity. Start light, then dig in with the palm of your hands, using circular motions.

2. Squeeze each toe, then move up the leg squeezing your Achilles tendon, calves, knees, and thighs. Be sure to intensify the pressure on tougher muscles, like your calves and quads.

3. Finally, to ease cramped muscles, make a fist with your hand and drum your way up your legs, starting at your feet. Vary the intensity, but be gentle with yourself.

Refresh Your Senses Scalp Oil

HEADACHES, MENTAL FOG, STRESS, TENSION • TOPICAL • **MAKES ABOUT 2 OUNCES**

Safe for ages 6+; not safe for pregnant or nursing women

Anyone who has had their hair washed at the salon knows the best part of the entire visit is the moment the stylist massages your scalp. Scalp massages can stimulate hair growth, relieve tension, and even soothe headaches. This invigorating scalp oil will refresh your senses and rejuvenate your mind.

¼ **cup unrefined coconut oil, melted**

10 drops lavender essential oil

10 drops eucalyptus essential oil

5 drops frankincense essential oil

1. In a medium glass bowl, stir together the coconut oil and lavender, eucalyptus, and frankincense essential oils.

2. Pour the mixture into a clean Mason jar, label and date your creation, and store in a cool, dark location.

Swap it out: *Eucalyptus essential oil has a high cineole content and, therefore, its use should be avoided around small children and pregnant or nursing women. To make this blend kid and pregnancy approved, substitute rosalina essential oil for the eucalyptus essential oil in this recipe.*

Invigorating Scalp Massage

1. Massage the Refresh Your Senses Scalp Oil into your scalp, starting from the sides and working your way toward the front and back of your head.

2. Gently massage your entire head using your fingertips, then grab fistfuls of your hair at the roots and gently tug from side to side, keeping your knuckles as close to your scalp as possible.

3. Squeeze your temples using the heels of your hands and gently massage your temples using slow, wide, circular motions.

Headache Helper Roll-On

ENERGY, HEADACHES, STRESS, TENSION • TOPICAL • **MAKES ABOUT 2 OUNCES**

Safe for ages 6+; not safe for pregnant or nursing women

Headaches are a common issue when you are overstimulated, tired, and stressed. Peppermint essential oil is one of my favorite oils to reach for when I am plagued by a headache or migraine. This Headache Helper Roll-On combines peppermint essential oil with lavender and eucalyptus to reduce inflammation, open the sinuses, and soothe tension to target the pain.

1. In a ⅓-ounce glass roll-on bottle, combine the peppermint, eucalyptus, lavender, and sweet marjoram essential oils.

2. Add fractionated coconut oil to fill the bottle. Place the rollerball cap on and gently swirl the bottle to mix. Label and date your creation.

3. To use, roll this blend onto your temples, the back of your neck, and between your brows on your forehead. Take care to avoid getting this blend into your eyes.

5 drops peppermint essential oil

2 drops eucalyptus essential oil

2 drops lavender leaf essential oil

1 drop sweet marjoram essential oil

Fractionated coconut oil, to fill

Helpful hint: *Oftentimes, headaches are symptoms of larger issues, including dehydration, magnesium deficiency, lack of sleep, caffeine addiction, and even hunger. I always suggest addressing these issues to find the source of your headaches. It never hurts to drink a full glass of water whenever you feel a headache coming on.*

Union Valley Headache Pressure Point

Before starting, apply the Headache Helper Roll-On as directed in step 3 of the recipe (this pressure point exercise can also be done without the roll-on).

1. The Union Valley pressure points are located on both hands, in the webbing between your thumb and index finger. Start by firmly pinching this area between your thumb and index finger of your opposite hand for 10 seconds.

2. Using your thumb, stroke small circles on the Union Valley pressure point in one direction for 10 seconds, then switch directions and stroke small circles for another 10 seconds.

3. Repeat this process with your opposite hand.

Tired Feet Massage Oil

HEADACHES, MUSCLE ACHES, STRESS, TENSION • TOPICAL • **MAKES ABOUT 2 OUNCES**

Safe for ages 2+ (use half the amount of essential oils for children 2 to 4 years of age)

No matter where you carry your stress and tension in your body, taking care of your feet can relieve pressure everywhere. This rejuvenating massage oil will reduce inflammation, soothe tired feet, and even relieve tension and headaches.

¼ cup carrier oil of choice

20 drops rosalina essential oil

10 drops lavender essential oil

10 drops sweet marjoram essential oil

1. In a medium glass bowl, stir together the carrier oil and rosalina, lavender, and sweet marjoram essential oils.

2. Pour the mixture into a lotion pump bottle (or other preferred container). Label and date your creation and store in a cool, dark location.

Helpful hint: *When your feet are tired after a long day, soak them in an Epsom salt footbath before using this massage oil for the most luxurious, relaxing end to a busy day.*

Magic Foot Massage

1. Start by applying the Tired Feet Massage Oil to lubricate your feet for massage. Start the massage by rubbing the base of your little toe.

2. Move to the next toe and continue rubbing. Apply gentle pressure to the flesh between your little toe and the one next to it.

3. Move on to your middle toe and massage, stretch and pull the toe in a circular motion. Do the same for the rest of your toes.

4. Using your knuckles, firmly press them into the ball of your foot, kneading it as you would bread.

5. Gently apply pressure to both sides of your heel, slightly below the ankle, using your fingertips or the palms of your hands. Rub around your ankle in a clockwise motion.

6. Finally, knead and squeeze your calf muscle to help relieve tension. Repeat this on your other foot.

Kick That Crick Neck Relief Oil

HEADACHES, MUSCLE ACHES, STRESS, TENSION • **TOPICAL** • **MAKES ABOUT 2 OUNCES**

Safe for ages 2+ (use half the amount of essential oils for children 2 to 4 years of age)

As a person living with severe scoliosis, waking up with a painful crick in my neck is a very common occurrence for me. Over the years, I have fine-tuned the pain relief oil I use to help kick that crick in the neck to the curb. This is a simple version of the oil that I use when neck pain is a problem.

1. In a medium glass bowl, stir together the olive oil and peppermint, lavender, and sweet marjoram essential oils.

2. Pour the mixture into a lotion pump bottle (or other preferred container). Label and date your creation and store in a cool, dark location.

¼ cup olive oil

20 drops peppermint essential oil

10 drops lavender essential oil

10 drops sweet marjoram essential oil

Swap it out: *CBD-infused oil has become a favorite of mine when it comes to muscle pain and a stiff neck. If nothing else is touching the pain in your neck, substitute a CBD-infused carrier oil for olive oil in this recipe and find the pain relief you are looking for.*

Note: *If you choose to try CBD-infused oil, since this blend is being applied topically and not being ingested, it shouldn't have any contraindications for use. However, it is always best to consult with your doctor before adding anything new to your regimen.*

Trapezius Muscle Massage

For this massage, you need a sock, a tennis ball, and a comfortable place to sit or lie down. Place the tennis ball in the sock and place the sock diagonally across your back. The toe should drape over your right shoulder and the open end should fall under your left arm.

1. Apply pressure to the tennis ball using one (or all) of these techniques:

   * Pull the sock tight and move the tennis ball around your back for a light massage.
   * Lean back in a chair or place your back against the wall. Let the tennis ball apply pressure to specific points, or move it around to create pressure.
   * Lie on the ground and move your body on the ball.

2. Switch the sock and tennis ball to massage the opposite side.

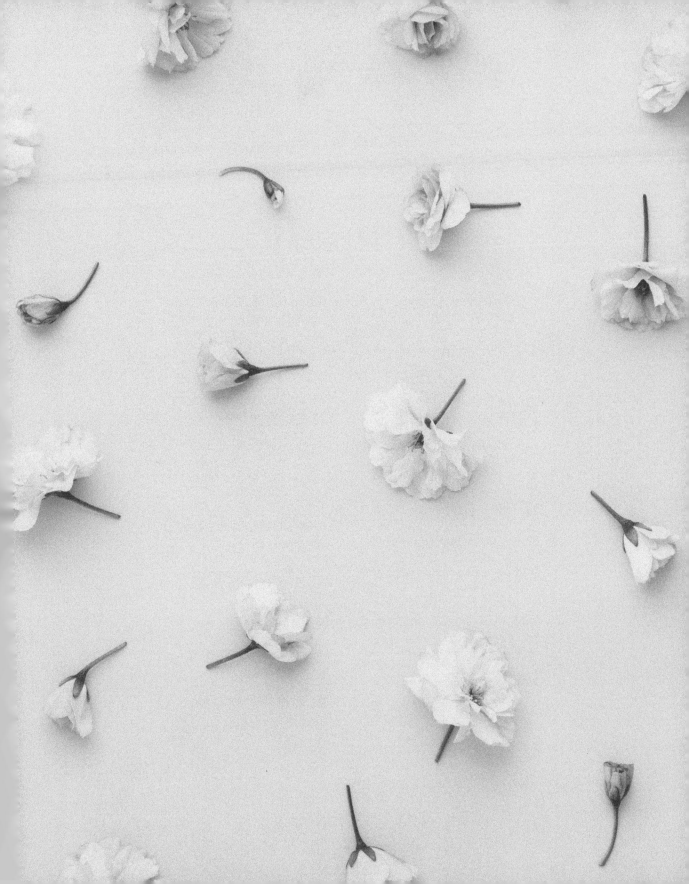

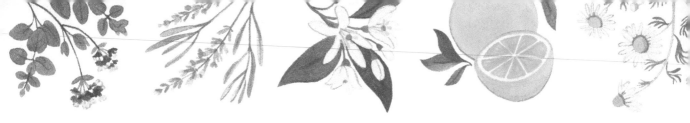

8

Remedy

Calm Your Squirrel Diffuser Blend

ANXIETY, CONCENTRATION, MENTAL FOCUS, NERVOUS TENSION • AROMATIC • **MAKES ½ OUNCE**

Safe for ages 2+

When mental fog is blocking you from focusing on the tasks at hand, essential oils can help clear your head and calm an overactive mind. Studies have shown Atlas cedarwood, lavender, and vetiver help improve cognitive function, increase focus, and calm overstimulated nerves.

1. In a dark glass dropper-top essential oil bottle, combine the lavender, Atlas cedarwood, grapefruit, vetiver, and frankincense essential oils. Gently swirl the bottle to mix. Label and date your creation.

2. Add 8 to 10 drops to a diffuser and diffuse throughout the room in 30-minute intervals (30 minutes on, 30 minutes off).

Swap it out: *This essential oil blend can also be applied topically in an aromatherapy roll-on bottle or used as a massage oil if diluted following the Traditional Dilution Chart (page 10).*

1 teaspoon lavender essential oil

¾ teaspoon Atlas cedarwood essential oil

¾ teaspoon grapefruit essential oil

¼ teaspoon vetiver essential oil

¼ teaspoon frankincense essential oil

Clear the Fog Aromatherapy Roll-On

COGNITIVE FUNCTION, CONCENTRATION, MENTAL FATIGUE, MENTAL FOCUS •
AROMATIC, TOPICAL • **MAKES ⅓ OUNCE**

Safe for ages 6+; not safe for pregnant or nursing women

It can be difficult to focus when your brain is cloudy from stress and anxiety, but essential oils can help clear the fog and boost your brainpower. This uplifting blend combines cedarwood and basil with the citrus aroma of bergamot and grapefruit to help you perform at your best even when you're stressed.

1. In a ⅓-ounce glass roll-on bottle, combine the bergamot, Atlas cedarwood, grapefruit, and basil essential oils.

2. Add fractionated coconut oil to fill the bottle. Place the rollerball cap on and gently swirl the bottle to mix. Label and date your creation.

3. To use, roll the blend onto the nape of your neck, behind your ears, and on your palms. Gently massage it in.

4. Cup the palms of your hands over your nose and mouth and breathe in the fog-clearing scent.

5 drops bergamot essential oil

2 drops Atlas cedarwood essential oil

2 drops grapefruit essential oil

1 drop basil essential oil

Fractionated coconut oil, to fill

Swap it out: *Grapeseed oil is my favorite carrier oil to use in perfume oils. It's not greasy, sinks into the skin quickly, and carries the scent longer than other oils. For the longest-lasting scent, substitute grapeseed oil for fractionated coconut oil in this recipe.*

Don't Overthink It Aromatherapy Inhaler

ANXIETY, FEAR, NERVOUS TENSION, RACING THOUGHTS • AROMATIC • **MAKES 1 TREATMENT**

Safe for ages 2+

It can be difficult to shut down the anxious thoughts that get in the way of accomplishing everyday tasks. Take a break from overthinking everything and inhale this bright, uplifting blend. Close your eyes, clear your mind, and inhale.

1. In a small glass bowl, combine the lavender, grapefruit, Roman chamomile, and blue tansy essential oils.

2. Using tweezers, add the personal aromatherapy inhaler wick (the cotton pad) to the bowl and roll it around until it's soaked up all the essential oils.

3. Using tweezers, transfer the wick to the inhaler tube. Close the tube and label and date your creation.

4. Inhale, as needed.

10 drops lavender essential oil

3 drops grapefruit essential oil

3 drops Roman chamomile essential oil

3 drops blue tansy essential oil

1 clean wick for personal aromatherapy inhaler

Swap it out: *Both coriander and rosalina essential oils have similar linalool content to lavender essential oil, making them great substitutes when you want to change up this recipe. Substitute either coriander or rosalina essential oils for the lavender essential oil in this recipe.*

Immune Support Diffuser Blend

IMMUNE SUPPORT, RESPIRATORY SUPPORT, SLEEP SUPPORT • AROMATIC • **MAKES ½ OUNCE**

Safe for ages 2+

Stress, anxiety, depression, and even insomnia can negatively affect your immune system, putting you at risk for illness. This blend combines the antibacterial and antiviral properties of lavender, frankincense, and rosalina essential oils to provide immune system support when you need it most.

1. In a dark glass dropper-top essential oil bottle, combine the lavender, frankincense, lemon, rosalina, and fir needle essential oils. Gently swirl the bottle to mix. Label and date your creation.

2. Add 8 to 10 drops to a diffuser and diffuse throughout the room in 30-minute intervals (30 minutes on, 30 minutes off).

Swap it out: *This essential oil blend can also be applied topically in an aromatherapy roll-on bottle or used as a massage oil if diluted following the Traditional Dilution Chart (page 10).*

1 teaspoon lavender essential oil

¾ teaspoon frankincense essential oil

¾ teaspoon lemon essential oil

¼ teaspoon rosalina essential oil

¼ teaspoon fir needle essential oil

Curb the Cravings Aromatherapy Inhaler

DEPRESSION, EMOTIONAL EATING, SADNESS • AROMATIC • **MAKES 1 TREATMENT**

Safe for ages 2+

Emotional eating is a common coping mechanism, but it's not a healthy response to stress and anxiety. Essential oils can be used to retrain your brain and curb cravings so you can eat food for physical, not emotional, sustenance.

1. In a small glass bowl, combine the grapefruit, coriander, sweet orange, and lime essential oils.

2. Using tweezers, add the personal aromatherapy inhaler wick (the cotton pad) to the bowl and roll it around until it's soaked up all the essential oils.

3. Using tweezers, transfer the wick to the inhaler tube. Close the tube and label and date the inhaler.

4. Inhale, as needed.

10 drops grapefruit essential oil

3 drops coriander essential oil

3 drops sweet orange essential oil

3 drops lime essential oil

1 clean wick for personal aromatherapy inhaler

Swap it out: *Sweet smelling essential oils can help train your brain to curb your cravings. If you don't have lime essential oil on hand, use lemon or even vanilla essential oil in this recipe instead.*

Cool Vibes Vapor Rub

IMMUNE SUPPORT, MUSCLE ACHES, RESPIRATORY SUPPORT, SLEEP •
AROMATIC, TOPICAL • **MAKES ABOUT 4 OUNCES**

Safe for ages 6+

When respiratory support is needed, eucalyptus essential oil is the most popular choice to help improve circulation and open the airways. This vapor rub will help you breathe deeply when you have shortness of breath, soothe inflamed airways, and support your immune system through illness.

1. In a medium pan over low heat, melt the coconut oil and beeswax.

2. Once melted, remove from the heat and stir in the eucalyptus, peppermint, lavender, and sweet marjoram essential oils.

3. Pour the mixture into a 4-ounce Mason jar and put it into the freezer for about 20 minutes to harden. Store with the lid on tight, labeled and dated, in a cool, dark location for up to 2 years.

4. Apply to your chest, back, and neck whenever better breathing is needed.

6 tablespoons unrefined coconut oil

2 tablespoons beeswax

50 drops eucalyptus essential oil

25 drops peppermint essential oil

15 drops lavender essential oil

15 drops sweet marjoram essential oil

Helpful hint: *This salve is multi-purpose and can be used to soothe sore muscles, an achy back, and even a headache.*

Anti-Nausea Aromatherapy Inhaler

GAS, MOTION SICKNESS, NAUSEA, UPSET TUMMY • AROMATIC • **MAKES 1 TREATMENT**

Safe for ages 6+; not safe for pregnant or nursing women

Nausea can strike at any time and for many reasons, including stress and anxiety. Studies have shown that essential oils, when inhaled, can dramatically reduce nausea and vomiting. This soothing blend combines the digestive properties of mint, ginger, and chamomile to help calm your tummy.

1. In a small glass bowl, combine the peppermint, Roman chamomile, spearmint, and ginger essential oils.

2. Using tweezers, add the personal aromatherapy inhaler wick (the cotton pad) to the bowl and roll it around until it's soaked up all the essential oils.

3. Using tweezers, transfer the wick to the inhaler tube. Close the tube and label and date the inhaler.

4. Inhale, as needed.

Swap it out: *Mint is well known for its ability to soothe nausea, but peppermint essential oil is rich in menthol, making it not the best option for babies and pregnant women. To make this recipe for children or pregnant women, substitute coriander essential oil for the peppermint essential oil in this recipe.*

10 drops peppermint essential oil

3 drops Roman chamomile essential oil

3 drops spearmint essential oil

3 drops ginger essential oil

1 clean wick for personal aromatherapy inhaler

Tummy Tamer Roll-On

ACID REFLUX, GAS, INDIGESTION, NAUSEA • AROMATIC, TOPICAL • **MAKES ⅓ OUNCE**

Safe for ages 2+

Whether you are suffering from illness or anxiety, this roll-on will ease your tummy woes. In the case of an upset stomach, indigestion, or gas, apply this roll-on to the abdomen to help tame your tummy.

1. In a ⅓-ounce glass roll-on bottle, combine the Roman chamomile, spearmint, ginger, and petitgrain essential oils.

2. Add fractionated coconut oil to fill the bottle. Place the rollerball cap on and gently swirl the bottle to mix. Label and date your creation.

3. To use, roll the blend onto your abdomen, massaging in a gentle circular motion.

Swap it out: *If you are making this blend for adults and children over the age of 6, peppermint essential oil can be substituted for the spearmint essential oil in this recipe.*

5 drops Roman chamomile essential oil

2 drops spearmint essential oil

2 drops ginger essential oil

1 drop petitgrain essential oil

Fractionated coconut oil, to fill

Energizing Diffuser Blend

Safe for ages 6+

Everyone can use a little energizing boost every now and then. This energizing diffuser blend will give you a boost if you feel your energy drop. This blend is also great to help get your mind and body going in the morning.

1. In a dark glass dropper-top essential oil bottle, combine the sweet orange, peppermint, lemon, eucalyptus, and geranium essential oils. Gently swirl the bottle to mix. Label and date your creation.

2. Add 8 to 10 drops to a diffuser and diffuse throughout the room in 30-minute intervals (30 minutes on, 30 minutes off).

Swap it out: *You can also apply this blend topically in an aromatherapy roll-on bottle or used as a massage oil if diluted following the Traditional Dilution Chart (page 10).*

1 teaspoon sweet orange essential oil

¾ teaspoon peppermint essential oil

¾ teaspoon lemon essential oil

¼ teaspoon eucalyptus essential oil

¼ teaspoon geranium essential oil

Wake Up and Go Energizing Body Wash

BRAIN FOG, ENERGY, MENTAL FATIGUE, MENTAL FOCUS •
AROMATIC, TOPICAL • **MAKES 16 OUNCES**

Safe for ages 2+ (use half the amount of essential oils for children 2 to 4 years of age)

Homemade body wash is one of my favorite ways to soap up in the shower. It's very easy to make, takes no time at all, and can easily be adapted to what you have on hand. This energizing body wash is the perfect way to start your day with a little more pep in your step.

1. In a 16-ounce bottle with a flip-top lid, combine the castile soap, vegetable glycerin, hemp seed oil, and sweet orange, grapefruit, spearmint, and rosalina essential oils.

2. Seal tightly and gently flip the bottle up and down to combine. Label your creation and store in your bathtub.

3. To use, squirt a quarter-size amount of body wash onto a loofah or washcloth and wash as you would with store-bought body wash. Rinse clean after washing.

Awesome addition: *For an extra-luxurious moisturizing body wash, substitute 2 tablespoons argan oil for 2 tablespoons of the hemp seed oil in this recipe.*

1 cup liquid castile soap

½ cup vegetable glycerin

½ cup hemp seed oil

50 drops sweet orange essential oil

50 drops grapefruit essential oil

20 drops spearmint essential oil

20 drops rosalina essential oil

Keep the (Blood) Pressure Low Aromatherapy Inhaler

ANXIETY, CIRCULATION, STRESS, TENSION • AROMATIC • **MAKES 1 TREATMENT**

Safe for ages 2+

High blood pressure is an extremely common problem in people experiencing stress, anxiety, and tension. Aromatherapy is an effective complementary treatment to lower blood pressure, decrease cortisol levels, and even support healthy circulation.

1. In a small glass bowl, combine the bergamot, lavender, ylang-ylang, and melissa essential oils.

2. Using tweezers, add the personal aromatherapy inhaler wick (the cotton pad) to the bowl and roll it around until it's soaked up all the essential oils.

3. Using tweezers, transfer the wick to the inhaler tube. Close the tube and label and date the inhaler.

4. Inhale, as needed.

10 drops bergamot essential oil

3 drops lavender essential oil

3 drops ylang-ylang essential oil

3 drops melissa essential oil

1 clean wick for personal aromatherapy inhaler

Helpful hint: *This same essential oil blend can be used in your diffuser, too! Simply add it to your diffuser instead of the personal aromatherapy inhaler to help relieve feelings of tension throughout your home.*

Social Butterfly Aromatherapy Roll-On

FEAR, NERVOUS TENSION, SOCIAL ANXIETY, STAGE FRIGHT •
AROMATIC, TOPICAL • **MAKES ⅓ OUNCE**

Safe for ages 2+

Social anxiety can be debilitating. Don't let fear and anxiety keep you from experiencing your best life. This roll-on will help soothe your fears and bring you out of your cocoon so you can spread your wings.

1. In a ⅓-ounce glass roll-on bottle, combine the bergamot, rosalina, coriander, and lemongrass essential oils.

2. Add fractionated coconut oil to fill the bottle. Place the rollerball cap on and gently swirl the bottle to mix. Label and date your creation.

3. To use, roll the blend onto the nape of your neck, behind your ears, and on your palms. Gently massage it in.

4. Cup the palms of your hands over your nose and mouth and breathe in the cozy scents.

Swap it out: *Grapeseed oil is my favorite carrier oil to use in perfume oils because it is not greasy, sinks into the skin quickly, and carries the scent longer than other oils. For the longest-lasting scent, substitute grapeseed oil for the fractionated coconut oil in this recipe.*

5 drops bergamot essential oil

2 drops rosalina essential oil

2 drops coriander essential oil

1 drop lemongrass essential oil

Fractionated coconut oil, to fill

Monsters-B-Gone Room and Pillow Spray

FEAR, INSOMNIA, NIGHTMARES, RACING THOUGHTS • AROMATIC • MAKES ABOUT 4 OUNCES

Safe for ages 2+

When my son was a toddler, he was afraid of monsters in his room at night. To calm and soothe his fears and help relax his mind for sleep, I designed this Monsters-B-Gone spray. I sprayed it all over his bedroom to protect him from monsters, and the results were magnificent! That night he happily fell asleep without a care in the world.

1. In a 4-ounce spray bottle, combine the witch hazel and lavender, Roman chamomile, tangerine, and vanilla essential oils. Gently swirl the bottle to mix.

2. Add distilled water to fill the bottle.

3. Cover the bottle and label and date your creation.

4. To use, shake well. Spray the mist into the air and on furniture and bedding (pillows, blankets, sheets, mattresses, and bedroom curtains). Store in a cool, dark location.

¼ cup witch hazel

40 drops lavender essential oil

30 drops Roman chamomile essential oil

30 drops tangerine essential oil

15 drops vanilla essential oil

Distilled water, to fill

Swap it out: *For an even sweeter addition, substitute chamomile hydrosol for the water in this recipe. Chamomile hydrosol is a soothing hydrosol that can help calm your nerves during times of tension and worry.*

Calming the Child Roll-On

ANGER, OVERSTIMULATION, RESTLESS MIND, SLEEP ISSUES •
AROMATIC, TOPICAL • **MAKES ⅓ OUNCE**

Safe for ages 2+

Sometimes our busy world can be just as stressful for kids as it is for us. When tempers flare, it's often a reaction to overstimulation and emotional fluctuations. This sweet-scented blend is beloved by all because of its ability to promote tranquility and calm heightened emotions.

1. In a ⅓-ounce glass roll-on bottle, combine the mandarin, tangerine, lavender, and Roman chamomile essential oils.

2. Add fractionated coconut oil to fill the bottle. Place the rollerball cap on and gently swirl the bottle to mix. Label and date your creation.

3. To use, roll the blend onto nape of your neck, behind your ears, and on your palms. Gently massage it in.

4. Cup the palms of your hands over your nose and mouth and breathe in the cozy scents.

2 drops mandarin essential oil

2 drops tangerine essential oil

2 drops lavender essential oil

1 drop Roman chamomile essential oil

Fractionated coconut oil, to fill

Helpful hint: *This blend can help calm adults as well. When you feel your inner child starting to throw a tantrum, whip out this aromatherapy roll-on and give them a gentle dose of calming the child.*

Craving Kicker Aromatherapy Inhaler

ADDICTION, ANXIETY, CRAVINGS, IRRITABILITY • AROMATIC • **MAKES 1 TREATMENT**

Safe for ages 2+

A study from the medical journal *Drug and Alcohol Dependence* shows that inhaling black pepper essential oil in place of a cigarette can help drastically reduce the intensity of nicotine cravings. Though this essential oil blend is no "cure-all," it is designed to help relieve some of the cravings you might experience when trying to kick the smoking habit.

1. In a small glass bowl, combine the black pepper, bergamot, Roman chamomile, and grapefruit essential oils.

2. Using tweezers, add the personal aromatherapy inhaler wick (the cotton pad) to the bowl and roll it around until it's soaked up all the essential oils.

3. Using tweezers, transfer the wick to the inhaler tube. Close the tube and label and date the inhaler.

4. Inhale, as needed.

10 drops black pepper essential oil

3 drops bergamot essential oil

3 drops Roman chamomile essential oil

3 drops grapefruit essential oil

1 clean wick for personal aromatherapy inhaler

Helpful hint: *Although this inhaler was created to curb the urge to smoke, that is not its only purpose. This inhaler can also help to reduce food cravings. Inhale when you get a craving.*

Good Vibrations Mood Booster Body Spray

ANXIETY, DEPRESSION, SADNESS, STRESS • AROMATIC, TOPICAL • **MAKES ABOUT 4 OUNCES**

Safe for ages 2+ (use half the amount of essential oils for children 2 to 4 years of age)

Everybody needs some good vibrations in their life. Whether you want a mood boost or to smell like a delightful ray of sunshine, this spray will make your day brighter.

1. In a 4-ounce spray bottle, combine the witch hazel, aloe vera gel, vegetable glycerin, and the coriander, lavender, lemongrass, and ylang-ylang essential oils. Gently swirl the bottle to mix.

2. Add distilled water to fill the bottle. Cap the bottle and shake well. Label and date your creation.

3. To use, shake the mixture first, then spray it all over your body (avoiding your face) and clothing.

Swap it out: *Elevate this delightful body spray by adding lime peel hydrosol. Substitute lime peel hydrosol for water for a fresh, calming slice of heaven.*

¼ cup witch hazel

1 tablespoon aloe vera gel

1 teaspoon vegetable glycerin

20 drops coriander essential oil

20 drops lavender essential oil

10 drops lemongrass essential oil

5 drops ylang-ylang essential oil

Distilled water, to fill

Let It Go Aromatherapy Roll-On

ANGER, IRRITABILITY, NERVOUS TENSION, SADNESS • AROMATIC, TOPICAL • **MAKES ⅓ OUNCE**

Safe for ages 2+

When you need to bring more peace and calm into your life, the Let It Go Aromatherapy Roll-On will help calm nervous tension and soothe irritability.

1. In a ⅓-ounce glass roll-on bottle, combine the tangerine, blue tansy, lemon, and ylang-ylang essential oils.

2. Add fractionated coconut oil to fill the bottle. Place the rollerball cap on and gently swirl the bottle to mix. Label and date your creation.

3. To use, roll the blend onto the nape of your neck, behind your ears, and on your palms. Gently massage it in.

4. Cup the palms of your hands over your nose and mouth and breathe in the calming scent.

Helpful hint: *This blend doubles as a mood elevator when you are feeling blue—and as a delightful aphrodisiac, too!*

5 drops tangerine essential oil

2 drops blue tansy essential oil

2 drops lemon essential oil

1 drop ylang-ylang essential oil

Fractionated coconut oil, to fill

Temper Tamer Diffuser Blend

AGITATION, ANGER, IRRITABILITY, MOODINESS • AROMATIC • **MAKES ½ OUNCE**

Safe for ages 2+; not safe for pregnant or nursing women

When tempers flare, a calming tranquil environment can help put out the flames. This soothing diffuser blend can uplift spirits, soothe irritability, and even ease physical responses to anxiety.

1. In a dark glass dropper-top essential oil bottle, combine the bergamot, frankincense, lavender, Roman chamomile, and clary sage essential oils. Gently swirl the bottle to mix. Label and date your creation.

2. Add 8 to 10 drops to a diffuser and diffuse throughout the room in 30-minute increments (30 minutes on, 30 minutes off).

Swap it out: *This essential oil blend can also be applied topically in an aromatherapy roll-on bottle or as a massage oil if diluted following the Traditional Dilution Chart (page 10).*

1 teaspoon bergamot essential oil

¾ teaspoon frankincense essential oil

¾ teaspoon lavender essential oil

¼ teaspoon Roman chamomile essential oil

¼ teaspoon clary sage essential oil

Aunt Flo's Soothing Massage Oil

CRAMPS, FRAZZLED NERVES, HORMONAL FLUCTUATIONS, STRESS • TOPICAL • **MAKES ½ OUNCE**

Safe for ages 10+; not safe for pregnant or nursing women

When my least favorite aunt comes to town, I am always ready to combat the "gifts" she brings. I have experienced painful and emotional periods since I was a teenager. Not wanting to consume pills to ease the pain, I designed this soothing massage oil to help ease the pain, soothe frazzled nerves, and calm emotional meltdowns.

1. In a medium pan over low heat, melt the olive oil and beeswax together.

2. Once melted, remove from heat and add the clove, lavender, geranium, bergamot, clary sage, and ginger essential oils.

3. Pour the mixture into a 4-ounce Mason jar, label and date your creation, and put it into the freezer for about 20 minutes to harden.

4. Apply the oil to your abdomen, lower back, and thighs to reduce cramping, pain, and to soothe frazzled nerves.

6 tablespoons olive oil

2 tablespoons beeswax

30 drops clove essential oil

20 drops lavender essential oil

15 drops geranium essential oil

15 drops bergamot essential oil

10 drops clary sage essential oil

10 drops ginger essential oil

Awesome addition: *Arnica flowers and St. John's wort are herbs known for their anti-inflammatory and pain-relieving properties. In step 1, infuse 2 tablespoons dried arnica flowers and 2 tablespoons dried St. John's wort in the olive oil over low heat for 2 hours. Strain and continue with the recipe as directed.*

Libido Lift Diffuser Blend

NERVOUSNESS, STRESS, LIBIDO • AROMATIC • MAKES ½ OUNCE

Not safe for pregnant or nursing women, or children under 2

When stress and anxiety get to be too much, your libido may seem subdued or out of reach, but essential oils can help you set the mood and boost sexual desire. Libido Lifter Diffuser Blend was created with known aphrodisiac essential oils to help you get out of your head and into the mood.

1. In a dark glass dropper-top essential oil bottle, combine the sweet orange, lavender, cinnamon, clove, and vanilla essential oils. Gently swirl the bottle to mix. Label and date your creation.

2. Add 8 to 10 drops to a diffuser and diffuse throughout the bedroom 30 minutes before the romantic interlude takes place.

Helpful hint: *This blend can be used in a massage oil as well. Combine 1 ounce of your favorite carrier oil with 18 drops of this blend and have your partner massage your back, chest, legs, or feet.*

1 teaspoon sweet orange essential oil

¾ teaspoon lavender essential oil

¾ teaspoon cinnamon leaf essential oil

¼ teaspoon clove essential oil

¼ teaspoon vanilla essential oil

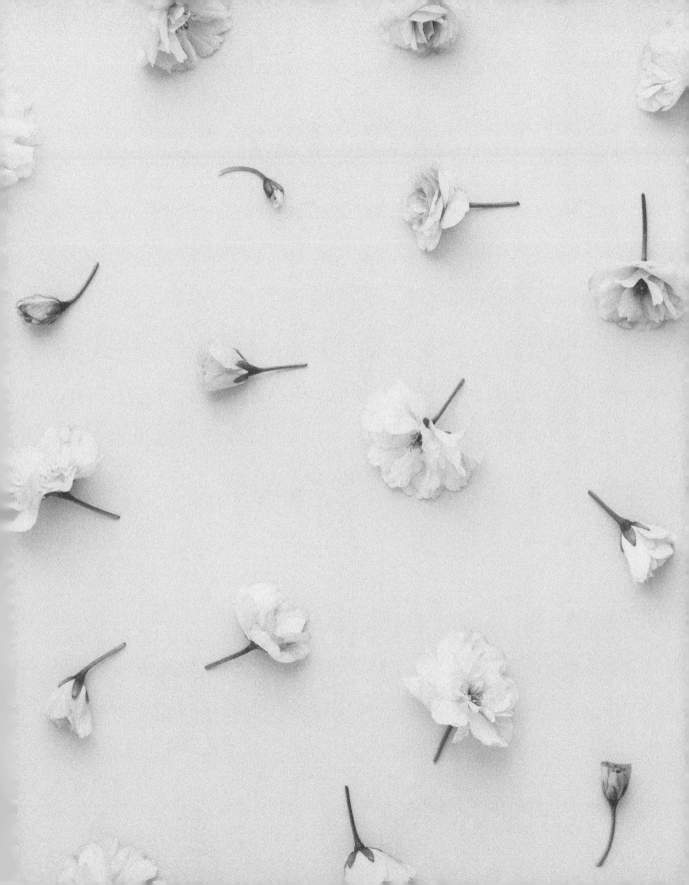

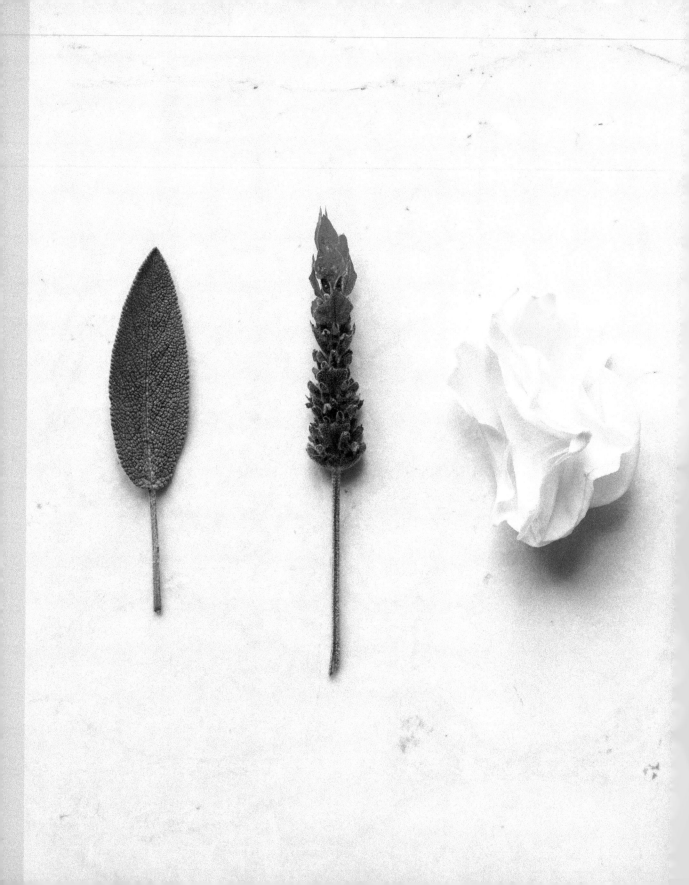

Resources

Whether you are just starting your aromatherapy journey or have spent years learning to use these oils, there are many great resources available to help you find aromatherapy schools, certified aromatherapists, and even where to purchase essential oils. Following are some of my favorite resources to help you grow as an aromatherapist and build your home apothecary.

Alliance of International Aromatherapists (www.alliance-aromatherapists.org)

This nonprofit alliance seeks to advance aromatherapy research, promote the responsible use of essential oils, and establish and maintain professional educational standards. You can find information on safety, research, registered aromatherapy schools, and more on their website.

Anthis, Christina. *The Beginner's Guide to Essential Oils: Everything You Need to Know to Get Started.* Emeryville: Althea Press, 2019.

If you are new to essential oils, this is the perfect book to get you started! My book is full of recipes for beauty, health, and home care.

Anthis, Christina. *The Complete Book of Essential Oils for Mama and Baby: Safe and Natural Remedies for Pregnancy, Birth, and Children.* Emeryville: Althea Press, 2017.

If you or someone you know is pregnant, nursing, or has children, my book is full of recipes and information on the safe use of essential oils at every stage and age.

Mountain Rose Herbs (www.MountainRoseHerbs.com)

One of my favorite places to shop for all my essential oil and herbal needs, Mountain Rose Herbs is a zero-waste–certified company that is an eco-friendly source for 100% certified organic herbs, essential oils, carrier oils, and all the other ingredients needed to make personal care items and cosmetics.

National Association for Holistic Aromatherapy (www.NAHA.org)

This member-based nonprofit association provides a wealth of aromatherapy knowledge, including scientific information, safety data, education resources, professional standards, and a list of certified aromatherapists.

Plant Therapy Essential Oils (www.PlantTherapy.com)

Plant Therapy is an affordable source for high-quality essential oils, carrier oils, and aromatherapy accessories. The company worked with Robert Tisserand to create KidSafe sets of essential oil blends.

Tisserand, Robert, and Rodney Young. *Essential Oil Safety: A Guide for Health, 2nd edition.* Philadelphia: Churchill Livingstone, 2013.

This updated and comprehensive book on safety standards for essential oils contains chemical profiles as well as safety data and recommendations.

References

Akhlaghi, M., G. Shabanian, M. Rafieian-Kopaei, N. Parvin, M. Saadat, and M. Akhlaghi. "Citrus Aurantium Blossom and Preoperative Anxiety." *Revista Brasileira de Anestesiologia* 61, no. 6 (2011): 702–12.

Alliance of International Aromatherapists. "Aromatherapy." https://www.alliance-aromatherapists.org/aromatherapy.

American Psychological Association. "Anxiety." 2019. www.apa.org/topics/anxiety/.

Bachir, Raho, and M. Benali. "Antibacterial Activity of the Essential Oils from the Leaves of *Eucalyptus Globulus against Escherichia Coli* and *Staphylococcus Aureus*." *Asian Pacific Journal of Tropical Biomedicine* 2, no. 9 (2012): 739–42. doi.org/10.1016/S2221-1691(12)60220-2.

Baser, K., and Gerhard Buchbauer, eds. *Handbook of Essential Oils: Science, Technology, and Applications*. 2nd edition. Boca Raton, FL: CRC Press, 2005.

Bensouilah, Janetta, and Philippa Buck. *Aromadermatology: Aromatherapy in Treatment and Care of Common Skin Conditions*. New York: Routledge, 2001.

Borges, Anabela, Ana Cristina Abreu, Carla Dias, Maria José Saavedra, Fernanda Borges, and Manuel Simões. "New Perspectives on the Use of Phytochemicals as an Emergent Strategy to Control Bacterial Infections Including Biofilms." *Molecules* 21, no. 7 (2016): 877. doi.org/10.3390/molecules21070877.

Buckle, Jane. *Clinical Aromatherapy Essential Oils in Healthcare*. 3rd edition. St. Louis, MO: Churchill Livingstone, 2014.

Catty, Suzanne. *Hydrosols: The Next Aromatherapy*. Rochester, VT: Healing Arts Press, 2001.

Chang, Kang-Ming, and Chuh-Wei Shen. "Aromatherapy Benefits Autonomic Nervous System Regulation for Elementary School Faculty in Taiwan." *Evidence-Based Complementary and Alternative Medicine*, 2011. doi.org/10.1155/2011/946537.

Choi, Seo Yeon, Purum Kang, Hui Su Lee, and Guen Hee Seole. "Effects of Inhalation of Essential Oil of Citrus Aurantium L. var. Amara on Menopausal Symptoms, Stress, and Estrogen in Postmenopausal Women: A Randomized Controlled Trial." *Evidence-Based Complementary and Alternative Medicine*, 2014. http://dx.doi.org/10.1155/2014/796518.

Clark, Demetria. *Aromatherapy and Herbal Remedies for Pregnancy, Birth, and Breast-feeding.* Summertown, TN: Book Publishing Company, 2015.

Clarke, Marge. *Essential Oils and Aromatics.* Seattle, WA: Amazon Digital Services, 2013.

Conrad, Pam, and Cindy Adams. "The Effects of Clinical Aromatherapy for Anxiety and Depression in the High-Risk Postpartum Woman: A Pilot Study." *Complementary Therapies in Clinical Practice* 18, no. 3 (2012): 164–68. doi.org/10.1016/j.ctcp.2012.05.002.

Da Silva, Gabriela L., Carolina Luft, Adroaldo Lunardelli, Robson H. Amaral, Denizar A. Da Silva Melo, Márcio V. F. Donadio, Fernanda B. Nunes, et al. "Antioxidant, Analgesic, and Anti-Inflammatory Effects of Lavender Essential Oil." *Anais da Academia Brasileira de Ciências* 87, no. 2 (2015): 1397–408. http://dx.doi.org/10.1590/0001-3765201520150056.

Deckard, A. "11 Proven Peppermint Essential Oil Benefits." *Healthy Focus*, May 27, 2016. https://healthyfocus.org/proven-peppermint-essential-oil-benefits.

Donaldson, Jill, Cynthia Ingrao, Diane Drake, and Emilou Ocampo. "The Effect of Aromatherapy on Anxiety Experienced by Hospital Nurses." *MedSurg Nursing* 26, no. 3 (2017): 201–6.

Effati-Daryani, Fattemeh, Sakineh Mohammad-Alizadeh-Charandabi, Mojgan Mirghafourvand, Moshen Taghizadeh, and Azam Mohammadi. "Effect of Lavender Cream with or without Foot-Bath on Anxiety, Stress, and Depression in Pregnancy: A Randomized Placebo-Controlled Trial." *Journal of Caring Sciences* 4, no. 1 (2015): 63–73. https://doi.org/10.5681/jcs.2015.007.

Fernandes Pimenta, Flavia Cristina, Mateus Feitosa Alves, Martina Bragante Fernandes Pimenta, Silvia Adelaide Linhares Melo, Anna Alice Figueiredo de Almeida, José Roberto Leite, Liana Clébia de Morais Pordeus, et al. "Anxiolytic Effect of Citrus Aurantium L. on Patients with Chronic Myeloid Leukemia." *Phytotherapy Research* 30, no. 4 (2016): 613–17. doi.org/10.1002/ptr.5566.

Fifi, Amanda C., Cara Hannah Axelrod, Partha Chakraborty, and Miguel Saps. "Herbs and Spices in the Treatment of Functional Gastrointestinal Disorders: A Review of Clinical Trials." *Nutrients* 10, no. 11 (2018): 1715. doi.org/10.3390/nu10111715.

Fißler, Maria, and Arnim Quante. "A Case Series on the Use of Lavendula Oil Capsules in Patients Suffering from Major Depressive Disorder and Symptoms of Psychomotor Agitation, Insomnia and Anxiety." *Complementary Therapies in Medicine* 22, no. 1 (2014): 63–9.

Fradelos, Evangelos, and Asimina Komini. "The Use of Essential Oils as a Complementary Treatment for Anxiety." *American Journal of Nursing Science* 4, no. 1 (2015): https://www.researchgate.net/publication/265715636_The_use_of_essential_oils_as_a_complementary_treatment_for_anxiety.

Franco, Lola, Thomas J. J. Blanck, Kimberly Dugan, Richard Kline, Geetha Shanmugam, Angela Galotti, Annelise von Bergen Granell, and Michael Wajda. "Both Lavender Fleur Oil and Unscented Oil Aromatherapy Reduce Preoperative Anxiety in Breast Surgery Patients: A Randomized Trial." *Journal of Clinical Anesthesia* 33 (2016): 243–49. http://dx.doi.org/10.1016/j.jclinane.2016.02.032.

Furlow, F. Bryant. "The Smell of Love." *Psychology Today*, March 1996.

Gattefossé, René-Maurice. *Gattefossé's Aromatherapy*. 2nd revised edition. Ebury Digital, 2012.

Gatti, Giovanni, and Renato Cajola. *The Action of Essences on the Nervous System*. Italy, 1923.

Hinton, Devon E., Thang Pham, Minh Tran, Steven A. Safren, Michael W. Otto, and Mark H. Pollack. "CBT for Vietnamese Refugees with Treatment-Resistant PTSD and Panic Attacks: A Pilot Study." *Journal of Traumatic Stress* 17, no. 5 (2004): 429–33. www.ncbi.nlm.nih.gov/pmc/articles/PMC2748790/.

Hirsch, Alan, and Jason Gruss. "Human Male Sexual Response to Olfactory Stimuli." *American Academy of Neurological and Orthopaedic Surgeons*, March 3, 2014. https://aanos.org/human-male-sexual-response-to-olfactory-stimuli/.

Inouye, Shigeharu, Toshio Takizawa, and Hideyo Yamaguchi. "Antibacterial Activity of Essential Oils and Their Major Constituents Against Respiratory Tract Pathogens by Gaseous Contact." *Journal of Antimicrobial Chemotherapy* 47, no. 5 (2001): 196–207. doi.org/10.1093/jac/47.5.565.

Kasper, Siegfried, Ion Anghelescu, and Angelika Dienel. "Efficacy of Orally Administered Silexan in Patients with Anxiety-Related Restlessness and Disturbed Sleep: A Randomized, Placebo-Controlled Trial." *Journal of European Neuropsychopharmacology* 25, no. 11 (2015): 1960–67. doi.org/10.1016/j.euroneuro.2015.07.024.

Keim, Joni, and Ruah Bull. *Aromatherapy & Subtle Energy Techniques: Compassionate Healing with Essential Oils*. Scotts Valley, CA: CreateSpace, 2015.

Khadivzadeh, Talat, Mona Najaf Najafi, Musumeh Ghazanfarpour, Morvarid Irani, Fatemeh Dizavandi, and Khatereh Shariati. "Aromatherapy for Sexual Problems in Menopausal Women: A Systematic Review and Meta-Analysis." *Journal of Menopausal Medicine* 24, no. 1 (2018): 56–61. doi.org/10.6118/jmm.2018.24.1.56.

Kia, Parisa Yavari, Farzaneh Safajou, MahnzaShahnazi, and Hossein Nazemiyeh. "The Effect of Lemon Inhalation Aromatherapy on Nausea and Vomiting of Pregnancy: A Double-Blinded, Randomized, Controlled Clinical Trial." *Iranian Red Crescent Medical Journal* 16, no. 3 (2014). www.ncbi.nlm.nih.gov/pubmed/24829772.

Knezevic, Peter, Verica Aleksic, Natasa Simin, Emilija Svircev, Aleksandra Petrovic, and Neda Mimica-Dukic. "Antimicrobial Activity of Eucalyptus Camaldulensis Essential Oils and Their Interactions with Conventional Antimicrobial Agents Against Multi-Drug Resistant *Acinetobacter Baumannii*." *Journal of Ethnopharmacology* 178 (February 3, 2016): 125–136. doi.org/10.1016/j.jep.2015.12.008.

Köse, E., M. Sarsilmaz, S. Meydan, M. Sönmez, I.Kus, and A. Kavakli. "The Effect of Lavender Oil on Serum Testosterone Levels and Epididymal Sperm Characteristics of Formaldehyde-Treated Male Rats." *European Review for Medical and Pharmacological Sciences* 15, no. 5 (2011): 538–42. www.ncbi.nlm.nih.gov/pubmed/21744749.

Koulivand, Pier Hossein, Maryam Khaleghi Ghadiri, and Ali Gorji. "Lavender and the Nervous System." *Evidence-Based Complementary and Alternative Medicine* 2013. doi.org/10.1155/2013/681304.

Lafta, Alexia. "How Our Sense of Smell Makes Us Fall in Love and Stay in Love." *Elite Daily*, June 29, 2015, www.elitedaily.com/dating/sense-of-smell-makes-us-love /1094795.

Lahmar, Aida, Ahmed Bedoui, Imen Mokdad-Bzeouich, Zaineb Dhaouifi, Zahar Kalboussi, Imed Cheraif, Kamel Ghedira, and Leila Chekir-Ghedira. "Reversal of Resistance in Bacteria Underlies Synergistic Effect of Essential Oils with Convention Antibiotics." *Microbial Pathogenesis* 106 (May 2017): 50–9. doi.org/10.1016 /j.micpath.2016.10.018.

Lawless, Julia. *The Encyclopedia of Essential Oils: The Complete Guide to the Use of Aromatic Oils in Aromatherapy, Herbalism, Health & Well-Being.* San Francisco: Conari Press, 2013.

Lee, Kyung-Bok, Eun Cho, and Young-Sook Kang. "Changes in 5-Hydroxytryptamine and Cortisol Plasma Levels in Menopausal Women after Inhalation of Clary Sage Oil." *Phytotherapy Research* 28, no. 11 (2014): 1599–1605. doi.org/10.1002/ptr .5163.

Lillehei, Angela S., and Linda L. Halcon. "A Systematic Review of the Effect of Inhaled Essential Oils on Sleep." *Journal of Alternative and Complementary Medicine* 20, no. 6 (2014): 441–51. doi.org/10.1089/acm.2013.0311.

Mechan, Annis O., Ann Fowler, Nicole Seifert, Henry Rieger, Tina Wöhrle, Stéphane Etheve, Adrian Wyss, et al. "Monoamine Reuptake Inhibition and Mood-Enhancing Potential of a Specified Oregano Extract." *British Journal of Nutrition* 105, no. 8 (2011): 1150–63. doi.org/10.1017/S0007114510004940.

Mojay, Gabriel. *Aromatherapy for Healing the Spirit: A Guide to Restoring Emotional and Mental Balance Through Essential Oils*. London: Gaia, 2005.

Morris, Edwin. *Scents of Time: Perfume from Ancient Egypt to the 21st Century*. New York: The Metropolitan Museum of Art, 1999.

Nagai, Katsuya, Akira Niijima, Yuko Horii, Jiao Shen, and Mamoru Tanida. "Olfactory Stimulatory with Grapefruit and Lavender Oils Change Autonomic Nerve Activity and Physiological Function." *Autonomic Neuroscience* 185 (2014): 29–35. doi.org /10.1016/j.autneu.2014.06.005.

Ni, Cheng-Hua, Wen-Hsuan Hou, Ching-Chiu Kao, Ming-Li Chang, Lee-Fen Yu, Chia-Che Wu, and Chiehfeng Chen. "The Anxiolytic Effect of Aromatherapy on Patients Awaiting Ambulatory Surgery: A Randomized Controlled Trial." *Evidence-Based Complementary and Alternative Medicine* 2013. http://dx.doi.org /10.1155/2013/927419.

Nunn, John F. *Ancient Egyptian Medicine*. London: British Museum Press, 1996.

Ostling, Michael. "Witches' Herbs on Trial." *Folklore* 125, no. 2 (July 2014): 179–201. doi:10.1080/0015587x.2014.890785.

Pertz, Heinz, Jochen Lehmann, René Roth-Ehrang, and Sigurd Elz. "Effects of Ginger Constituents on the Gastrointestinal Tract." *Planta Medica* 77, no. 10 (July 2011): 973–78. doi.org/10.1055/s-0030-1270747.

Price, Shirley. *Aromatherapy Workbook: A Complete Guide to Understanding and Using Essential Oils*. Thorsons, 2012.

Rose, Jed, and Frederique M. Behm. "Inhalation of Vapor from Black Pepper Extract Reduces Smoking Withdrawal Symptoms." *Drug and Alcohol Dependence* 34, no. 5 (1994): 225–29. doi.org/10.1016/0376-8716(94)90160-0.

Schnaubelt, Kurt. *The Healing Intelligence of Essential Oils: The Science of Advanced Aromatherapy*. Rochester, VT: Healing Arts Press, 2011.

Seenivasan, Prabuseenivasan, Jayakumar Manickkam, and Ignaciumuthu Savarimuthu. "In Vitro Antibacterial Activity of Some Plant Essential Oils." *BMC Complementary and Alternative Medicine* 6, article no. 39 (2006): 196–207. doi.org/10.1186/1472 -6882-6-39.

Sienkiewicz, Monika., Anna Głowacka, Edwrad Kowalczyk, Anna Wiktorowska-Owczarek, Marta Jóźwiak-Bębenista, and Monika Łysakowska. "The Biological Activities of Cinnamon, Geranium, and Lavender Essential Oils." *Molecules* 19, no. 12 (2014): 20929–40. doi.org/10.3390/molecules191220929.

Srivastava, Janmejai K., Eswar Shankar, and Sanjay Gupta. "Chamomile: A Herbal Medicine of the Past with a Bright Future (Review)." *Molecular Medicine Reports* 3, no. 6 (2010): 895–901. doi.org/10.3892/mmr.2010.377.

Stea, Susanna, Alina Beraudi, and Dalila De Pasquale. "Essential Oils for Complementary Treatment of Surgical Patients: State of the Art." *Evidence-Based Complementary and Alternative Medicine* 2014. http://dx.doi.org/10.1155/2014/726341.

Valnet, Jean. *The Practice of Aromatherapy: Classic Compendium of Plant Medicines and Their Healing Properties*. London: Ebury Digital, 2012.

Worwood, Valerie Ann. *The Fragrant Mind: Aromatherapy for Personality, Mind, Mood, and Emotion*. Novato, CA: New World Library, 1996.

Worwood, Valerie Ann. *Scents & Scentuality: Essential Oils & Aromatherapy for Romance, Love, and Sex*. Novato, CA: New World Library, 1999.

Yap, Polly Soo Xi, Beow Chin Yiap, Hu Cai Ping, and Swee Hua Erin Lim. "Essential Oils, A New Horizon in Combating Bacterial Antibiotic Resistance." *The Open Microbiology Journal* 8 (2014): 6–14. doi:10.2174/1874285801408010006.

Yap, Polly Soo Xi, Swee Hua Erin Lim, Cai Ping Hu, and Beow Chin Yiap. "Combination of Essential Oils and Antibiotics Reduce Antibiotic Resistance in Plasmid-Conferred Multidrug-Resistant Bacteria." *Phytomedicine* 20, nos. 8–9 (2013): 710–13. doi.org/10.1016/j.phymed.2013.02.013.

Index

Acknowledgments

I find it funny how my life mirrored the feelings of this book while writing it. In an ironic twist of fate, I found myself full of anxiety and stress during the writing process because of all the mishaps along the way.

I would like to thank my "partner in crime," Clint Hill, for helping me through the entire process. When my laptop broke, you gave me your computer. When I was so overwhelmed with work piling up that tears fell, you reminded me I could do this *and* make time for myself. I can't imagine writing this book without you! Frankly, I can't imagine living this life with anyone else! You are my person and I love you with all my heart and soul!

I would really like to thank my mom and dad for their constant support and belief that I can accomplish anything I set my mind to.

Finally, I would like to thank all the wonderful people at Callisto who worked really hard to make this book happen. Samantha Barbaro, you have been a wonderful editor to work with, and I am forever grateful for your support and tireless efforts to help me reach my deadlines.

About the Author

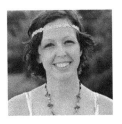 Christina Anthis is a single mother, bestselling author, and the blogger behind *The Hippy Homemaker*. As a committed do-it-yourselfer trained in aromatherapy and herbalism, she is devoted to helping others make safe and natural health and homecare products with essential oils. Christina, her son, and her partner, Clint, make their home in North Texas.

CPSIA information can be obtained
at www.ICGtesting.com
Printed in the USA
LVHW070102060220
645964LV00010B/22